CU00688359

Contents

Contents

About the author

The author Daniel Lannister has been involved in the health industry for over 25 years. He is a practitioner of common sense and has used his wealth of knowledge and experience in the health field to broaden people's minds.

His research into cancer has been ongoing for many years after having first-hand experience of family members being diagnosed with this disease.

He has personally helped many people to ask pertinent questions when considering options to fight cancer and has encouraged them to adopt a common sense approach to this disease.

By empowering others to challenge medical practitioners, Daniel has enabled people to see that they have options and can be in control on the journey back to health.

Many people like Kim, Mark and Mohammed have been shown that by using common sense in fighting their disease, they can come out the other side as a survivor.

These people are living proof that many options exist in the fight against cancer and like them; many others can successfully fight this disease.

*'I do not advise you
What you should believe
or not believe,
but I do advise you
that we all need to learn
as much as we can
about everything we can,
because one thing
I have learned in my life
is that most of what we have been taught
has been a lie.'*

William Cooper

Having received my cancer diagnosis in **February 2016** I was offered the conventional treatment options that all cancer patients are familiar with and decided to accept some of these. Alongside this, I was keen to gain a better understanding of the alternative natural and effective options that were available to me. The research I conducted gave me the confidence to implement natural treatments which I knew would help to empower my immune system. Once I understood the importance of the immune system in fighting cancer, I was clear as to what would help me to ensure I was in the best possible position to reverse the disease. It was important to me not to become a victim and hand control over my life to others. I wanted to take an active role in my recovery.

I was given the news that my cancer had been successfully reversed in **March 2018**.

This book 'Cancer and common sense' is an easy to understand pocket guide for everyone facing cancer and wanting to establish a common sense approach to this disease whether as a patient, or caring for someone with cancer. It is a great guide to living a healthy life and to keeping your body in optimum shape for fighting off disease.

'I highly recommend this guide and the options explained throughout.'

Kim Collister,

Cancer Survivor

Liverpool

Foreword

I was diagnosed with lung cancer on April 1st 2009 and was informed that this had spread to the lymph nodes in my chest. I felt like my world was falling apart with my first thought being for my wife and 5 children.

On 14th May 2009 I commenced 3 months of chemotherapy and radiotherapy which quickly took its toll on my body. I lost almost 5 stone within 12 months. I was given a 3 month terminal prognosis.

By 2012, I had suffered with pneumonia twice. It was during the same year that I decided to look into natural remedies and how they may benefit me. I started using 'NATURAL PLANT OIL' and was able to discontinue the 36 pharmaceutical drugs I had been prescribed.

By 2014, my body was feeling and looking better. This continued on into 2015 when I felt like my mind, body and soul were much stronger. On 31st March 2016, I returned for my routine scan results to be informed that my tumour had reduced in size by 75%. Although my battle is ongoing, I am living proof that cancer is by no means a death sentence.

A positive mind-set has been the key to my success in the battle against cancer. This, alongside the natural therapies I have adopted into my lifestyle have ensured that I have been alive for much longer than the medical profession anticipated.

Empowerment of the immune system is paramount. Without my wife and children I would not be here today. Here's to many more years helping people to win their battle with cancer. The book 'Cancer and common sense' is a must read for any person fighting cancer or anyone helping someone who is. I can highly recommend it.

Mark Clements

Liverpool

Reversing cancer since 2009 and living life to the full.

Throughout this pocket guide we aim to describe simple and effective interventions for those diagnosed with cancer. Our guidance is based on a common sense approach with suggestions as to how you can be proactive in the fight against cancer. Whilst it would be impracticable for this guide to cover all possible approaches to fighting cancer, our aim is to present a broad overview of some of the tried and tested options available. This will form a solid foundation from which

point, you will then be equipped to make informed choices about the options you have. There is no blanket approach – each individual will find their own path and we recognise that not all options will be suitable for all readers. Ultimately it is your choice as to which options are best – you are in control.

The pocket guide is here to assist you along the way and should be used as a supportive tool in your journey. The advice found within these pages is by no means

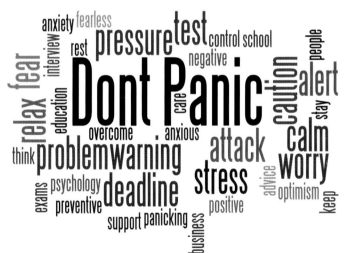

prescriptive and should be adapted for your own personal needs. At the end of each section you will find a summary of the information that has been presented. This will allow you to use the guide as a quick reference throughout your cancer journey and to take information from the guide at any time it is needed.

It is important to recognise that if chemotherapy, radiotherapy or surgery is what you decide is appropriate for you; this guide will be beneficial in preparing your body to ensure you are in the best possible position to undergo your treatment. In any given situation, the guide will support you through your journey and will enable you to make lifestyle changes that will empower your immune system to help your body to do what it is designed to do which is to fight all diseases including cancer.

Do not panic. Allow yourself the time and space to absorb all of the information that you have been given and to consider your options.

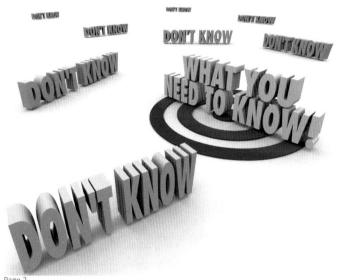

Do not feel under pressure to make decisions – a few days for example will make no significant difference to disease progression but will provide you with time to breath and process what is happening and how you wish to proceed.

Seek support from those around you but at the same time do not feel under duress to accept treatments just because others believe that they will be best for you. Only you have control over what happens.

Allow yourself to have an odd 'bad' day. This is to be expected. What is important is that you overcome the low points and move forward by refocussing on what you need to do to help yourself.

If you are a smoker, try to stop completely or at least reduce down. Start to focus on being in the best possible position to fight this disease.

Continue to exercise if this is already part of your regular routine. If it isn't, start with some gentle exercise that you are confident you will be able to maintain. This will help with the positive mind-set that you require at this difficult time.

Look at your diet – a few simple changes will reap huge rewards in the fight against cancer.

We aim to present the information in a way that is easily understood and will attempt to demonstrate the effectiveness of the adaptations to your lifestyle that we endorse. This will enable you to consider all of the information and to make the decisions that are right for you. We are not medical practitioners and have no desire to be. However, we are practitioners of common sense and have a wealth of experience in advising people how best to approach the fight against cancer. Our primary aim is to help people understand that the disease cancer is something that thousands of people worldwide reverse on a daily basis. Ultimately, they do this by using natural foods, herbs and plants which serve to empower our immune system and help it to function at its optimum. By practising strategies that are totally within your control, you will ultimately become more empowered. This will go a long way in your own journey to help your immune system to fight this disease and ultimately reverse it.

How has this happened to me?

The cells in the human body go through a repetitive process of production, maturation and death. If damage is caused to these cells and they cannot die naturally, clusters of damaged cells mixed with newly formed cells build up and potentially, tumours then develop. There are multiple predisposing factors which contribute to the chance of cancer developing. Some of these are not within our control – such as age, family history and gender. However, the lifestyle choices which we make can increase or decrease the risk of developing cancer.

Critically, it is a malfunction of the immune system that results in the development of cancer. This is the system that defends against disease and if this is compromised, there is

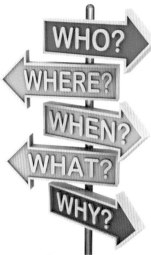

less protection against cancer development. In this guide we will explore many of the ways you can ensure that your immune system is functioning at its optimum level to protect you in future and to assist in fighting cancer.

Am I going to die from cancer?

It is important to remember that there are millions of people living with cancer and also many who have reversed their cancer. Untreated cancer will certainly result in death as the cancer cells invade key organs making survival impossible. Therefore, it is essential

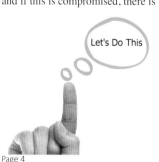

Let's Do This

that you make the right choices about how to treat your cancer. We will explore many of the options available to you which will give you the best chances of reversing your cancer. People reverse cancer on a daily basis.

How long can I live with cancer for?

This all depends on the type of cancer, how early your cancer is detected and what treatment choices you make. Untreated, cancer will spread and your prognosis will be poor. Therefore it is essential that you start your treatment early and focus on building your immune system up to ensure you have the best chances of longevity and of fighting this disease.

Can I reverse my cancer?

You can certainly take positive steps to help to fight cancer and reverse this disease. Throughout this guide you will find many of the treatment options that you can choose. Remember that many people worldwide reverse this disease every day.

What do I need to do to ensure that I am in the best health to undergo my treatment?

You need to empower your immune system to ensure that you are giving yourself the best chance of success. Some cancer treatments can take their toll on the body and will cause damage to healthy cells, not to mention the many side effects that these treatments can cause. Therefore, whatever treatment you choose, you must start by looking at your lifestyle and stop anything that could cause ill health. This guide will demonstrate how easy it is to boost your immune system and ensure you are in the best health possible.

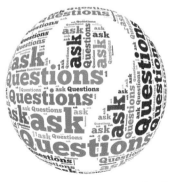

What do I need to eat to replace the vitamins, minerals and nutrients that are depleted during radiotherapy and chemotherapy?

It is known that conventional cancer treatments will deplete the vitamins, minerals and nutrients in the body. This is of obvious concern to any individual who is already ill and needs to build their immune system. A further reduction of vitamins, minerals and nutrients in an immune system that is already not functioning to its potential is dangerous. Therefore it is essential that you focus on maintaining an intake of foods rich in vitamins, minerals and nutrients to make strong health gains. This guide will show you what foods are needed and how you can ensure that you are feeding your body to boost your immune system.

Let's start at the beginning……

It is essential to start by looking at the basics which will form the foundation of your knowledge and will influence your approach to your fight against cancer. The essential

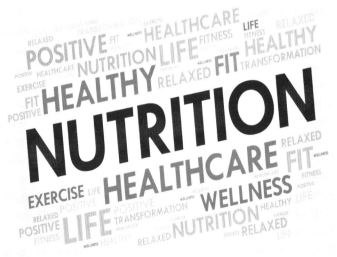

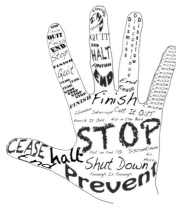

cancer

empower it to function at its optimum in fighting disease.

The human body is made up of a large amount of cells. Each of these cells is unique and has its own identity and function within the body. These cells have to discover how to interact and work together in order to maintain a healthy equilibrium within the body. Cancer cells are constantly forming in the body and our immune system has the ability to seek out these cells and destroy them before they take a strong hold within the body. However, tumours begin when more cancerous cells are being created in an overworked and depleted immune system. The immune system is too weak to be able to destroy these cancerous cells as a healthy immune system would be

factor to consider is that cancer is a disease of a compromised immune system. Our ultimate aim is to enable you to focus on working to strengthen your immune system. This will ensure that you are tackling cancer from its primary source which will in turn; enable you to have the reassurance that you are able to fight any possible reoccurrence of cancer in future. Common sense would tell us that we need to ensure that our immune system is prepared to fight any disease it is faced with. An effective immune system is developed and maintained by making certain that lifestyle habits feed the system to able to do. As a result of this, they are enabled to take hold in the body and cause destruction.

In an individual with a weakened immune system where cancer has developed, we must consider the notion of orthodox approaches which are so readily offered when cancer is detected. Radiotherapy, chemotherapy and surgical interventions come with side effects and cause further damage to the immune system. Therefore, the cancer that has developed due to a weakened immune system is then treated with an approach that weakens the immune system further. It is common sense to conclude that the likelihood of these interventions leaving the individual at high risk of recurrence of the disease is increased.

The traditional approaches to the treatment of cancer are known to damage and kill huge numbers of healthy cells within the body and can damage vital organs and affect the function of the lymphatic system. This results in the body being left in a compromised state. Unfortunately there is a high chance of disease regression over time when medically, the orthodox treatment appeared to have placed

the disease in remission. The orthodox approach does not allow for treating the root cause of cancer and certainly does not ensure that the body is left in an optimal state for fighting disease in the future.

Surgical approaches to cancer do not generally resolve the problem of cancer. A tumour is an uncontrolled growth of cells and is a symptom and side product of cancer. It is not the root cause of the disease and therefore, surgical intervention will allow for the removal of a tumour, but will not control the influx of cancerous cells that the weakened immune system cannot manage. If you imagine a tree that is cut down that is no longer visible above ground, under the surface the roots of the tree remain.

Cancer has the ability to migrate to different parts of the body and will grow without restriction. Problems are encountered when the tumour

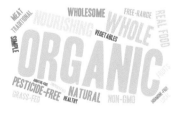

impinges on surrounding structures and their waste products may be toxic to the rest of the human body. This being so, they may at times interfere with the functions of organs such as the brain, lungs, liver and kidneys and this can result in complications and ultimately death.

Overcoming cancer is a process of reversing the conditions that enable the cancer to develop in the first instance. It is critical to note that cancer is a systemic imbalance - a problem with the entire system of the interrelated parts of the human body. This being so, appropriate options must involve a holistic approach focussing on the total environment of the body. This can be achieved by empowering the immune system with everything that is natural which will encourage it to gain strength and will help its effectiveness in fighting all diseases including cancer. It is essential to remember that this is happening every day for thousands of people worldwide who are empowering their immune system to fight this disease and to reverse cancer to the point where the cancer is completely eradicated.

IN BRIEF

You are in control.

The root cause of cancer lies in a weakened immune system.

Tackling cancer at its primary source is crucial.

The tumour is a by-product of cancer – not the root cause.

Treating the tumour will not reverse cancer.

Most orthodox approaches to cancer have side effects and will weaken the immune system further.

In strengthening your immune system, the body is better equipped to fight disease.

A holistic approach to cancer is necessary to address the systemic imbalance within the body.

A positive mind-set is needed to enable you to remain focussed and able to make the decisions that are right for you on your personal journey.

Cancer cannot be cured and therefore it can always return. It can however be reversed which happens every day for thousands of people.

Antioxidants are powerful substances which mostly come from the fruit and vegetables we consume. They have the ability to prohibit and prevent the oxidation of other molecules, therefore preventing cell damage within the body.

We will look at antioxidants in further detail in this section and will demonstrate the importance of antioxidants in maintaining your health.

One of the more obvious characteristics of plants is their wide range of bright colours. If you admire how food is presented, it is hard to beat the plate of fruits and vegetables with the variety of colours which are tempting and are extremely healthy. This link between brightly coloured vegetables and their exceptional health benefits has often been noted. It turns out that there is a beautiful scientifically sound story behind the correlation between colour and health. The colours of fruits and vegetables are derived from a variety of chemicals called antioxidants. These chemicals are almost exclusively found in plants and are only based in animal

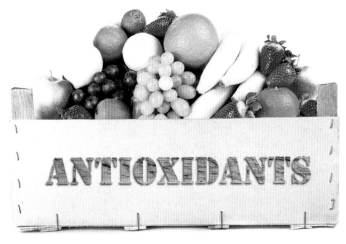

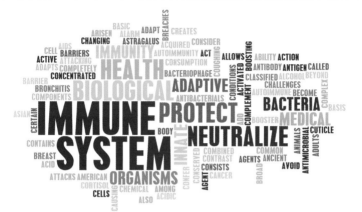

based foods to the extent that animals consume them and store small amounts in their own tissues. Living plants illustrate nature's beauty both in colour and chemistry. They take the energy of the sun and transform it into life through the process of photosynthesis. In this process, the sun's energy is first turned into simple sugars and then into more complex carbohydrates, fats and proteins. This complex process amounts to some high powered activity within a plant, all of which is driven by the exchange of electrons between molecules. Electrons are the medium of energy transfer. The site at which photosynthesis takes place is like a nuclear reactor. The electrons zoom around in the plant and convert the sunlight into chemical energy and this must be managed very carefully. If they stray from their rightful places in the process, they may create free radicals which can wreak havoc within the plant. It would be like the core of a nuclear reactor leaking radioactive materials that could be dangerous to the surrounding area.

So, how does the plant manage these complex reactions and protect itself against errant electrons and free radicals? It forms a shield around potentially dangerous reactions that sponges up these highly reactive substances. The shield is formed from antioxidants that intercept and scavenge electrons that may otherwise stray from their course. Antioxidants are usually coloured between the same chemical property that sponges up excess electrons and this also creates visible colours. Other antioxidants are colourless and these include chemicals such as ascorbic acid which is vitamin C and vitamin E which act as antioxidants in other parts of plants that need to be protected from the hazards of wayward electrons. What makes all of this relevant for us, is that we produce low levels of free radicals throughout our lifetime. Simply being exposed to the sun's rays, industrial pollutants and to improperly balanced nutrient intakes creates a background of unwanted free radical damage.

Free radicals are nasty and can cause our tissues to become rigid and limited in their function. This uncontrolled free radical damage is also part of the process that gives rise to cataracts, hardening of the arteries, cancer, emphysema,

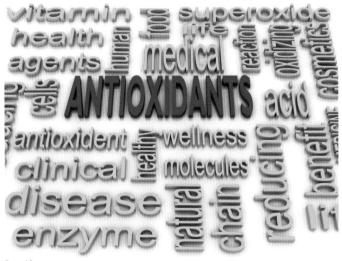

arthritis and many other ailments that develop with age. However, we do not naturally build shields to protect ourselves from free radicals as plants do. We do not carry out photosynthesis and therefore do not produce our own antioxidants. Fortunately though, the antioxidants from plants work within our bodies as they do in plants. Is it a wonderful harmony – the plants make the antioxidant shields and at the same time make them look incredibly attractive to eat. Then we as animals are attracted to the plants and in consuming them, benefit from their antioxidant shields. This is an incredible example of nature's wisdom.

IN BRIEF

Antioxidants are substances that protect cells from the damage caused by unstable molecules known as free radicals.

Free radical damage can contribute to causing cancer.

Antioxidants prevent free radical damage by interacting and stabilising them.

The body makes some of the antioxidants it uses to neutralise free radicals.

The body relies on external sources – primarily diet, to obtain the rest of the antioxidants it needs.

Antioxidants are abundant in fruits, vegetables, nuts and grains.

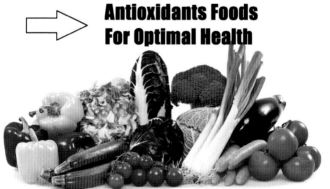

Antioxidants Foods For Optimal Health

Free radicals are created by oxidation and are molecules which have a missing electron. They seek out structures within the body from where they can neutralise an electron which in turn, leaves that structure seriously damaged.

We will look at free radicals in further detail in this section and will explain the damage free radicals can cause to our immune system on a daily basis.

Free radicals are everywhere. In order to understand what free radicals are, you need to know about human cells, where the tug of war between the free radicals and the antioxidants is played out every second of every day. Like everything else in the universe, cells are composed of smaller units called atoms. Each atom contains a centre or a nucleus that is surrounded by electrons. Two or more atoms may bind together by sharing electrons. Biological oxidisation, the process of making energy, involves moving electrons from one oxygen molecule to the next. However, sometimes an electron escapes and this free electron is called a free radical. Free radicals constantly form everywhere in the body at an astonishing rate. If these free radicals are not quickly trapped, they can cause a great deal

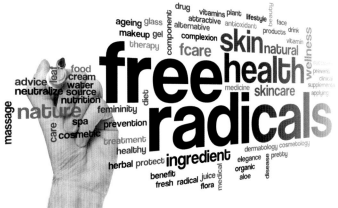

of damage. Free radicals can attack and oxidise DNA which is the genetic material that controls cell growth and development. This can increase the possibility of cancer.

One simple experiment that will demonstrate this is when you cut an apple in half. If this is left for a period of time, you will see the insides that have been exposed will have turned brown. That is free radical damage to the apple and although we are unable to see or smell the free radicals, we can see the damage they have caused.

However, the power of antioxidants can be demonstrated using the above experiment. If you squeeze lemon juice or lime juice on one half of the apple and leave it for a period of time, you will see that only half of the apple will be brown and the half with the lemon or lime juice on it will be as it was when it was cut. That is the power of vitamin C which is an antioxidant and is assisting in neutralising the free radical damage caused to the apple. Vitamin C is found in abundance in lemons and limes.

In summary, this demonstrates the need to have as much antioxidant

content in your daily diet. This can be found in the form of natural fruits and vegetables. Putting a consistent sufficient amount of antioxidants into your body will aid in neutralising the free radical damage that is constantly occurring inside and outside the body every second of every single day.

IN BRIEF

Free radical damage is constantly occurring inside and outside the body.

Free radicals can attack and oxidise DNA and therefore increase the risk of cancer developing.

Antioxidants neutralise free radical damage.

Antioxidants are found in real organic natural food. It is imperative that we have as much antioxidant content in our diets as possible.

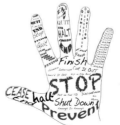

The Immune System

The immune system is the body's natural defence against all diseases including cancer and is made up with cells, proteins, tissues and organs. To function properly, the immune system must be able to detect these pathogens and be able to distinguish between them and the organisms own healthy tissue.

The immune system has the ability to recognise and remember millions of different infection-causing organisms and will produce secretions and cells to link to these and eradicate them. When the immune system receives the alert to the presence of a threat from invading microbes it responds to ensure that no damage occurs. It is therefore essential that it is empowered with the ingredients it requires to function effectively – namely vitamins, minerals, nutrients and cannabinoids.

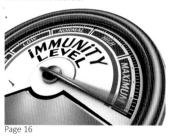

One of the important cells involved in the body's immune response are white blood cells which are also known as leucocytes. There are two types of leucocytes – phagocytes and lymphocytes. Phagocytes are able to pass through blood vessel walls into the surrounding tissue and move towards pathogens. They then either chew up the invading organisms or they release an enzyme which destroys them. Lymphocytes work by identifying disease-causing bacteria and either release antibodies or signal to other cells within the immune system so that the pathogen can be destroyed.

When the body is under attack, white blood cells along with other immune system cells flood to the area to assist in the destruction of harmful substance to prevent illness.

The immune response also operates to ensure that our bodies remain free from cancer cells. Millions of new cells are produced in our bodies on a daily basis and some of these will have faults or defects which may mean that they have the potential to become cancerous. The immune system has the ability to detect these damaged cells and can destroy them before they develop further. This is

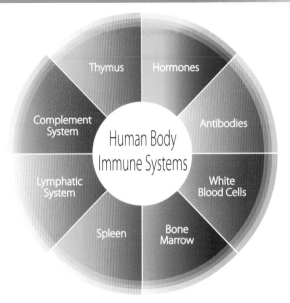

possible if the immune system is fully functioning and is empowered to do the job it is meant to do. If this quality control system fails, a faulty cell can go undetected and will then multiply and potentially wreak havoc.

The immune system functions better when it is protected from environmental attacks and is boosted by adopting healthy living strategies. Lack of sleep, unhealthy eating, sedentary lifestyle and chronic stress can all contribute towards weakening the immune system. Once the immune system is depleted, bacteria, toxins and viruses are able to overwhelm the body which in turn causes illness. The immune system is complex and to function well it requires harmony and balance. Just like any fighting force, the immune system marches on its stomach. Healthy nutritional intake and ensuring your body is not deficient in any of the vitamins and minerals it requires is essential to an empowered immune system.

Throughout this guide we will show you how to empower your immune system as this is essential for you in your fight against cancer. All of the lifestyle advice and options link back to the immune system which demonstrates the importance of empowering this complex system.

IN BRIEF

The immune system is a complex system comprising of cells, proteins tissues and organs.

It is the bodies defence mechanism against pathogens and protects us from illness and disease.

White blood cells work by identifying an invading pathogen and trigger a series of events to ensure that these are destroyed.

Cancerous cells can be detected by the immune system at an early stage to prevent them causing damage.

Ensuring that the immune system is empowered is vital to the prevention and fight against cancer.

Poor nutrition, lack of sleep, no exercise, exposure to pollution and increased stress will all impact on how effectively your immune system is able to function.

An already depleted immune system will require attention and your focus must be to build this up to ensure you give yourself the best possible outcome.

Intelligent eating habits are paramount. We need to feed the immune system and not feed the disease.

Immune system

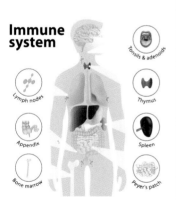

Tonsils & adenoids

Lymph nodes

Thymus

Appendix

Spleen

Bone marrow

Peyer's patch

The endogenous cannabinoid system — named for the plant that led to its discovery — is one of the most important physiological systems involved in establishing and maintaining human health. Endocannabinoids and their receptors are found throughout the body: in the brain, organs, connective tissues, glands, and immune cells.

With its complex actions in our immune system, nervous system, and virtually all of the body's organs, endocannabinoids are literally a bridge between body and mind. By understanding this system, we begin to see a mechanism that could connect brain activity and states of physical health and disease.

Cannabis is a naturally growing plant and has remained a source of controversy throughout its history. From debates on its medicinal value and legalisation to concerns about dependency and schizophrenia, cannabis (marijuana, pot, hashish, bhang, etc.) is a hot button for politicians and pundits alike. Fundamental to understanding these discussions is how cannabis affects the mind and body, as well as the body's cells and systems.

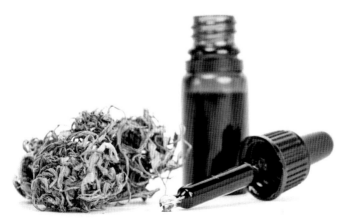

How can something that stimulates appetite also be great for relieving pain, nausea, seizures, and anxiety? Whether its leaves and buds are smoked, baked into pastries, processed into pills, or steeped as tea and sipped, cannabis affects us in ways that are sometimes hard to define. Not only are its many facets a fascinating topic, but because they touch on so many parts of the brain and the body, their medical, ethical, and legal ramifications are vast.

The intercellular signalling molecules, their receptors, and synthetic and degradative enzymes from which cannabis gets its powers had been in place for millions of years by the time humans began burning the plants and inhaling the smoke. Despite records going back over 4,000 years that document medicinal uses of cannabis, no one knew how it worked until 1964. That was when Yechiel Gaoni and Raphael Mechoulam reported that the main active component of cannabis is tetrahydrocannabinol (THC). THC, referred to as a "cannabinoid" (like the dozens of other unique constituents of cannabis), acts on the brain by muscling in on the intrinsic neuronal signalling system, mimicking a key natural player, and basically hijacking it for reasons best known to the plants. Since the time when exogenous cannabinoids revealed their existence, the entire natural complex came to be called the "endogenous cannabinoid system" or "endocannabinoid system" (ECS)

Back in the 1990s scientists were trying to understand how tetrahydrocannabinol (THC), the psychoactive substance in the cannabis plant, elicits its effect on the body. What they uncovered was a complex network of receptors (CB1) in the brain and central nervous system that were a perfect fit for the THC molecule.

Soon after another type of receptor (CB2) was discovered in the immune system, gut and many of the body's major organs. But that was only part of the puzzle. The hunt was on to find out whether the body produced its own cannabis-like chemicals, and with the identification of the first endocannabinoid Anandamide, they had their answer.

Scientists have realised that the endocannabinoid system fine-tunes most of our vital physiological functions, which in turn brings balance to everything from sleep, appetite, pain, inflammation, memory, mood and even reproduction. The system ensures that all sections are working

harmoniously maintaining a balance between the body and mind

Therefore the endocannabinoid system is an essential part of the body's immune system and is vital to ensure we remain healthy.

As the function of the endocannabinoid system is to bring balance to the body, it makes sense that activity within it is elevated in the presence of illness. This increase in activity demonstrates how the

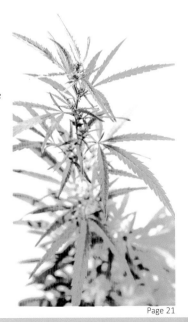

endocannabinoid system is making every effort to maintain harmony within the body.

The discovery of the endocannabinoid system has given a greater insight into why and how cannabis is beneficial in the treatment of illness and disease. The cannabis plant is one of the most pharmacologically active plants on earth and contains in excess of 400 active chemical ingredients. The unique active components of cannabis are cannabinoids, which are found alongside active chemicals called terpenoids and flavonoids. These components work in unison to provide a variety of therapeutic benefits to the body.

The two main cannabinoids from the cannabis plant that are of significant medical interest are

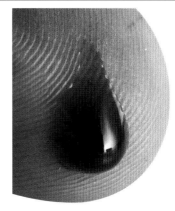

tetrahydrocannabinol (THC) and cannabidoil (CBD). Both of these interact with the body through the endocannabinoid system and their chemical make-up is similar to the body's own cannabinoids. However, CBD and THC have distinct differences in how they interact with the endocannabinoid system and therefore, the effects they have are different.

The human body was designed for cannabinoids as these are the substances that play a crucial role in the protection of cells against disease. They are also vital in the empowerment of the immune system, protection of the brain and nervous system and contribute to

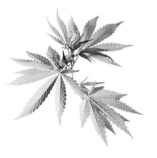

reducing pain and inflammation. One prime example as to the importance of cannabinoids is the discovery that human breast milk naturally contains the same cannabinoids found in the cannabis plant which have a vital role in human development. These cannabinoids in breast milk stimulate the suckling process in the new-born and provide them with a desire to eat. New born babies who are breast fed receive an abundance of cannabinoids that trigger hunger and promote their growth and development.

In recognising the importance of the endocannabinoid system, it is then possible to gain an understanding as to how to stimulate and support this complex system to maintain the balance in the body's immune and central nervous system. It plays a vital role in maintaining a healthy body and can decrease pain and inflammation levels, help to fight cancer and prevent neurodegenerative diseases to name a few. The potential in using this complex system for the benefit of maintaining health is great.

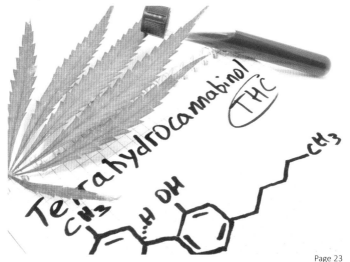

Endocannabinoid system

The endocannabinoid system is considered by some to be the most important physiologic system involved in establishing and maintaining human health.

This system helps to regulate the body's cell cycles, organ functions and nervous system and acts as a link between the cerebral function and physical health and disease.

It involves a complex system of cell receptors and corresponding molecules.

When the body creates neurotransmitters for the endocannabinoid system, they are picked up by specialised cannabinoid receptors that sit on the cells surface.

This works like a lock and key would – kick-starting a response to aid the body to achieve homeostasis despite external influences.

The human body was designed for cannabinoids as these are the substances that play a crucial role in the protection of cells against disease.

The discovery of the endocannabinoid system has given a greater insight into why and how cannabis is beneficial in the treatment of illness and disease.

Cannabis contains 2 main cannabinoids – THC and CBD.

THC and CBD have distinct differences in how they interact with the endocannabinoid system and therefore, the effects they have are different.

This is a natural plant that grows in the ground and many countries throughout the world understand the importance of this for medicinal purposes.

Dr Raphael Mechoulam is the pioneering scientist who discovered the THC cannabinoid and its importance within the human body.

Dr Mechoulam recognised that the THC interacts with the largest receptor system in the human body – The Endocannabinoid System.

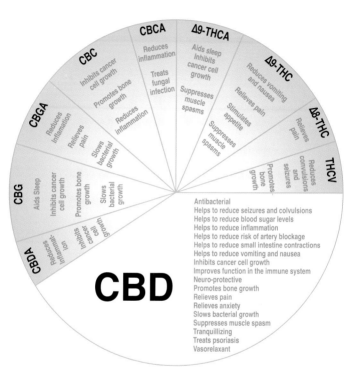

CBD

Antibacterial
Helps to reduce seizures and colvulsions
Helps to reduce blood sugar levels
Helps to reduce inflammation
Helps to reduce risk of artery blockage
Helps to reduce small intestine contractions
Helps to reduce vomiting and nausea
Inhibits cancer cell growth
Improves function in the immune system
Neuro-protective
Promotes bone growth
Relieves pain
Relieves anxiety
Slows bacterial growth
Suppresses muscle spasm
Tranquillizing
Treats psoriasis
Vasorelaxant

I**ntelligent eating habits are an essential component in the fight against all diseases including cancer. However, this is one area that has largely been ignored or dismissed when it comes to options.**

Until recent years, modern medicine has ignored the link between diet and disease. Instead, scientists have focussed on the discovery of the "magic bullets" which would wipe disease off the planet. There is no doubt that these modern developments have vastly improved our health but they may have given the false impression that no matter how serious the disease, the answer would be discovered in a well-equipped lab. The emphasis on high tech solutions for common health problems diminished the importance of lifestyle and healthy eating in the maintenance of health.

By the end of World War 2, people who were concerned about nutrition and health were considered to be food faddists at best or health nuts at worst. Fast food outlets offering highly processed, high fat foods were the rage. Hamburgers, chicken nuggets and French fries were "in". Fresh fruits and vegetables were out. Diet was considered so unimportant that few medical schools even offered courses in nutrition. It is essential to note that when a student attends medical school, the focus is on medicine and nutrition does not factor into the training schedule. Although doctors offer lip service to healthy eating, few understood what this actually entailed. At the same time, despite the increased medical knowledge, heart disease and cancer were becoming epidemic in the United States of America and Western Europe.

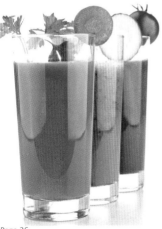

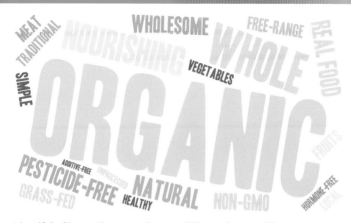

A handful of innovative researchers recognised this and began to look for reasons for this increase in disease. What was particularly striking was that this wasn't the case in other parts of the world. Numerous studies demonstrated that people living in less affluent countries where diet was rich in wholegrains and unprocessed fruits and vegetables had significantly lower rates of cancer and heart disease than in the wealthier and more advanced nations. Initially, many mainstream scientists dismissed these findings as purely coincidental or that some populations may be genetically prone to the development of different diseases. When scientists took a closer look at these studies, they found that certain foods appeared to protect against disease. There was no denying that people who ate an abundance of plant foods were healthier and lived longer than those who ate the traditional western diet. For the first time, these plant foods were studied using the same state of the art techniques that had previously been used only for the most cutting edge research. In labs around the world, scientists began to isolate particular chemicals in fruits and vegetables and commonly used spices, principally garlic and turmeric.

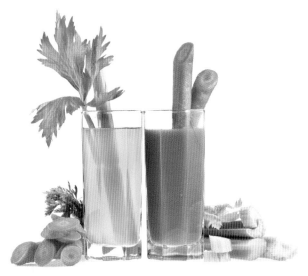

It was found that foods contained a wide array of protective compounds called phytochemicals, many of which were antioxidants. There are literally hundreds of phytochemicals which offer unique benefits. For example, the cruciferous vegetables such as broccoli have special chemicals that stimulate the production of anticancer compounds in the body. Soya beans are rich in isoflavones which are hormone like compounds that help to fight cancer. Citrus fruits contain a cancer fighting oil in their skin. The more that was found about fruits and vegetables, the more apparent it became that food was powerful medicine and from this research, we have learnt several important lessons.

First and foremost, there is no substitute for a healthy, well-balanced diet. Supplements can help enhance the health benefits of food but they are unable to do the job alone. Many of the important phytochemicals are in the pigments of plants, for example dark green leafy vegetables have different phytochemicals to those found in orange and yellow vegetables and therefore it is essential that we eat an assortment of brightly coloured vegetables daily so we can be assured that we are getting a full range of phytochemicals. Fresh whole fruits and vegetables are your best option. Although juice contains vitamins and minerals, only the whole fruit or vegetable contains fibre. Ideally you should also eat the skin of the fruit or vegetable as it is a wonderful source of nutrients. Many people are concerned about pesticides, insecticides and waxes used on produce to retain colour and freshness and these can be avoided by buying organic produce from a reputable source but be sure to scrub your produce thoroughly in hot water prior to consumption.

Bear in mind that there is no magic formula. There are many different phytochemicals in just one piece of fruit or vegetable and therefore it is impossible to say which is most important. In fact it is possible that a variety of phytochemicals work alongside each other or together to produce their effects. This being said, intelligent eating habits and understanding the power of food is a major piece of the puzzle in empowering your immune system as fruits and vegetables are all necessary to provide vitamins, minerals, nutrients and antioxidants to the body. It may help to consider just a small variety of foods and their benefits to enable you to understand the importance of a healthy diet to you in your fight against disease.

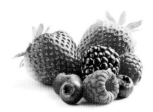

Berries can help to improve the condition of your skin and aid in the slowing down of the ageing process. They are beneficial in the fight against chronic health disorders and are proven to have a positive effect on memory. The consumption of berries can help reduce the risk of developing certain cancers. They are high in fibre and rich in antioxidants.

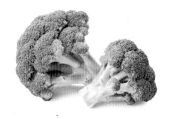

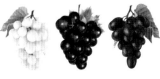

Grapes help in reducing anxiety and hypertension. This fruit is known to assist in the reduction of the risk of lung, prostate, colon, oesophageal, pancreatic, endometrial and oral cancers due to the antioxidants they contain.

Broccoli is known to assist in improving circulation as it is rich in iron. It will help to maintain a healthy heart and bones and can reduce cholesterol levels. Broccoli is a powerful antioxidant which helps in the fight against cancer and is rich in copper, fibre, potassium and vitamins K, B6, C and E.

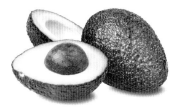

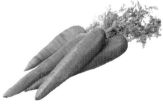

Avocados assist in the absorption of nutrients from vegetables and fruits, as well as helping to reduce cholesterol and improve the health of the heart. It contains fibre, nutrients and monounsaturated fatty acids.

Carrots can aid improvement in your thought process and eyesight because they contain a group of pigments which protect you against free radical damage. Carrots are rich in vitamin K, C, A, B8, iron and potassium.

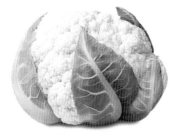

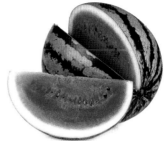

Cauliflower will help to boost the health of the heart and contains anti-inflammatory properties. One serving of this powerful vegetable will provide over 70% of the recommended daily intake of vitamin C. It is abundant in riboflavin, potassium, magnesium, vitamin K, thiamine and manganese.

Melon will help in the removal of toxins from the body and will assist in maintaining hydration. It has high water content and is an excellent alkaline food source.

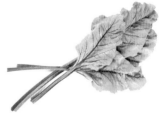

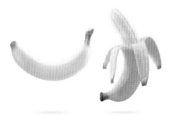

Swiss chard helps the heart and helps to regulate blood sugar levels. It helps the body to prevent virus as well as harmful bacteria and free radicals. It is the best source of alkali from all known foods.

Bananas have the ability to help to regulate the blood sugar levels in the body as well as helping to protect the heart and improve digestion. Bananas are rich in fibre as well as potassium, manganese, vitamin B and magnesium.

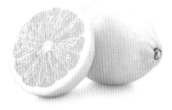

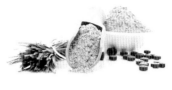

Lemons can be of benefit in the reduction of risk of stroke as well as in the treatment of kidney stones. Lemons contain vitamin E, A, C, B6 and many essential minerals such as zinc, calcium, potassium, copper and riboflavin. Lemons can assist in the fight against cancer and have anti-hypertensive properties.

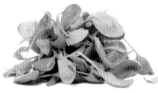

Spinach can help with the elimination of free radicals as well as improve memory and maintain a healthy heart. It is rich in antioxidants and is low in fat and cholesterol. Spinach contains vitamin A, C, K, B6, magnesium, potassium, calcium, zinc and iron.

Chlorella helps to cleanse the liver, gallbladder, kidneys and skin from alcohol, pesticides, heavy metals and other toxins.

This is merely a selection and another book could be written on this topic alone.

How powerful is food?

To test the power of dietary interventions to prevent DNA damage, scientists often study chronic smokers. Researchers rounded up a group of long term smokers and asked them to consume 25 times more broccoli than the average individual. In other words, a single stalk a day compared to broccoli avoiding smokers. The broccoli eating smokers suffered over 40% fewer DNA mutations in their blood stream over 10 days. Is this simply because the broccoli boosted the activity of the detoxifying enzymes in their livers which help to clear carcinogens before they made it to the smoker's cells? No. Even when the DNA was extracted from the subject's bodies and exposed to a known DNA damaging chemical, the genetic material from the broccoli eaters demonstrated significantly less damage. This suggests that eating vegetables such as broccoli may make you more resilient at a subcellular level. It is not correct to think that by eating a stalk of broccoli before smoking a packet of cigarettes is going to completely erase the cancer causing effects of the cigarette smoke as it won't. However, whilst trying to quit, consumption of vegetables such as broccoli, cabbage and cauliflower will help. The benefit of the broccoli family vegetables does not stop there. Whilst breast cancer is the

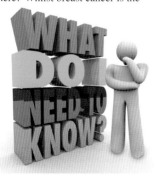

most common internal cancer among American women, lung cancer is actually their number 1 killer. Over 85% of women with breast cancer are still alive 5 years after diagnosis but the numbers are reversed when it comes to lung cancer. Over 80% of women die within 5 years of lung cancer diagnosis. Approximately 90% of these deaths are due to metastasis of the cancer to other parts of the body. Certain compounds in broccoli may have the potential to supress this spread of cancer.

In a 2010 study, scientists laid down a layer of human lung cancer cells in a petri dish and cleared a swath down the middle. Within 24 hours, the cancer cells had crept back together and within 30 hours the gap had closed completely. When the scientists dripped some cruciferous vegetable compounds onto the cancer cells, the cancer creep was stunted.

Yale University researchers followed over 500 women with non-Hodgkin's Lymphoma and found that those who consumed three or more servings of vegetables per day had over 40% improvement in survival rate over those who ate less or none at all.

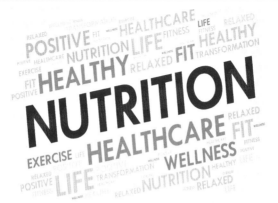

It is imperative to remember that healthy dietary interventions such as an increase in vegetable consumption have no disadvantages. This approach can therefore be added in to the treatment methods chosen by the individual. Consuming vegetables will have a huge impact on the empowerment of the immune system and will ultimately benefit your fight against cancer.

IN BRIEF

Food is essential in the fight against all diseases, including cancer.

There is no substitute for a healthy, well-balanced diet.

Protective compounds called phytochemicals are found in many foods.

Intelligent eating habits and understanding the power of food is critical.

Consumption of organic fruit and vegetables will empower your immune system.

Remember that there are no side effects to increasing your intake of fruit and vegetables.

There is a huge amount of literature debating whether vegetables are best eaten raw or cooked. Firstly we must remember the importance of eating vegetables and what this can do for your immune system. So it would make sense to assume that introducing vegetables into your diet- regardless of the preparation methods used is going to be more beneficial than not eating any vegetables at all.

It is obvious that how food is prepared will depend on what you will gain from eating it. Where cancer is concerned, our ultimate aim is to gain maximum benefit

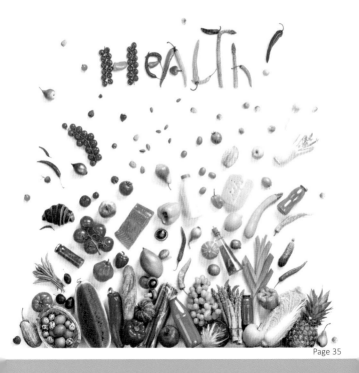

from the approaches we adopt so we need to look into the effects food preparation will have on the gains we will get. Nutrition in food can be diminished through processing (cutting, chopping or mashing), cooking or heating. Additionally, nutrients can be 'washed out' of the food during cooking processes that involve water.

Some nutrients, like vitamin C, are destroyed during the cooking process while other nutrients will become more absorbable after the cooking process. Cooked carrots for example, will give you approximately six times the amount of vitamin A in comparison to raw ones. On the flip side of this,

steamed broccoli will have approximately 10% less vitamin C than raw broccoli. Whilst cooked tomatoes will lose some of their vitamin C, the cooking process actually boosts the availability of the antioxidant lycopene.

Overall, this is very dependent on the volume of vegetables you are consuming throughout the day. The majority of literature available suggests eating vegetables raw which we will look into in more detail. Raw consumption prevents the destruction of enzymes and loss of food value although it is understandable that this approach is not suited to each individual.

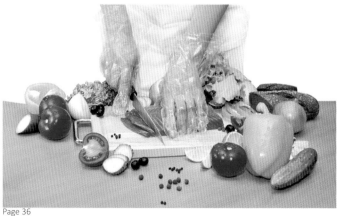

Firstly we need to begin with an explanation of the basics of a raw organic diet, the benefits this has and how you can make this adaptation to your lifestyle. This type of diet is focussed on the consumption of fresh, whole, unrefined, living plant-based foods which are fruits, vegetables, leafy greens, nuts and seeds. The raw food diet is based on the notion that these food groups are consumed in their natural state, without cooking or steaming to ensure that consumption of the highest nutritional value is gained.

The main benefit of the raw food approach is that you stop feeding your body with toxic residue that it must deal with which in turn will leave it free to cleanse and heal itself. The raw diet eliminates constipation, and the transit time of waste matter shortens to 24 hours or

less, which avoids the build-up of toxaemia from the recycling of toxins from the colon.

Learning how to eat a raw food diet properly takes time, patience, and effort. Most people find it challenging to adapt to a true raw food diet because the taste buds are accustomed to the excitement of salt, sugar and spices. Initially, it is common to miss those familiar tastes when they are no longer part of the daily diet. However, most people see the exchange for good health and longevity as a more favourable option. It is true that the taste buds will adapt and they develop an appreciation for the taste of sweet, fresh fruits and vegetables.

It is a common misconception that it is impossible to get all of our required nutrients from fruit and vegetables. However, the very best quality vitamins, mineral, antioxidants, enzymes, co-enzymes,

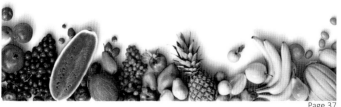

Raw Food Approach

fibre, water, protein, carbohydrates and fats are derived from these food sources. They are viewed as complete nutritional packages and have the ability to be the provider of everything that the body requires to function. Of all food sources, fruit is the richest in vitamins and water and second richest in minerals and fibre. Vegetables and leafy greens are richest in minerals and fibre and second richest in vitamins and water. The other two nutrient groups, proteins and fats, are needed in smaller quantities; so, while fruits and vegetables are not high in protein and fat content, they still remain their ideal source. All nutrients come in the proper proportions and ratios that the body can utilize optimally. No man-made vitamin tablet or other supplement can compare with nature's handiwork. Essentially, fruits supply nutrients in quantities that most closely approximate human nutritional needs and vegetables come in second place.

Applying heat to food provides no nutritional benefit and may be detrimental to the person ingesting the cooked food. However as mentioned previously, there are

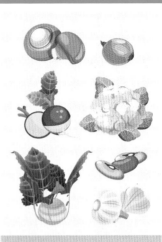

WHITE

 Immune system

 Protection of stomach

 Low cholesterol

 Healthy heart

 Healthy gut

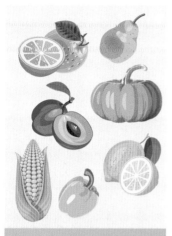

YELLOW

 Low cholesterol

 Healthy heart

 Healthy joints

 Eye protection

 Preventing cancer

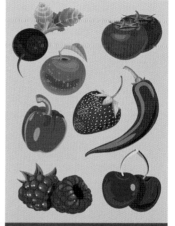

RED

 Healthy heart

 Healthy blood vessels

 Skin protection

 Cellular rejuvenation

 Preventing cancer

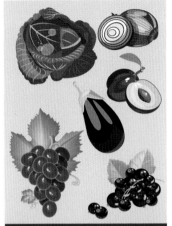

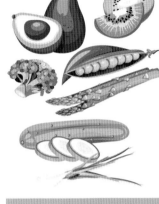

PURPLE

 Healthy heart

 Healthy blood vessels

 Improve your memory

 Cellular rejuvenation

 Protecting of the urogenital system

GREEN

 Protection of stomach

 Healthy bones

 Eye protection

 Immune system

 Preventing cancer

instances where, by heating food, certain nutrients are more easily released, like lycopene from tomatoes. However, this ignores the hundreds of other nutrients in that heated tomato that were damaged or destroyed and assumes that more of a specific nutrient is better.

Many foods that are cooked would otherwise be unappetizing or inedible to humans, such as meats and grains, thus bypassing sensory safeguards that would normally protect the body from ingestion of unnatural and unhealthy substances.

Studies have shown that the immune system often reacts to the introduction of cooked food into the bloodstream the same way it does to foreign pathogens such as bacteria, viruses, and fungi. Cooking food denatures the proteins, carcinogizes the fats, and caramelizes the carbohydrates. Most other nutrients are damaged, deranged or destroyed by the heating process, leaving mostly empty calories.

One way of consuming food in its raw state would be to make smoothies. This is a very simple and effective way to ensure that you gain the most benefit from the foods that you consume. Try some of the recipes below as a start. Unless stated, add all of the ingredients for your selected recipe to a blender and blend until smooth.

Green Smoothie

1 cup of coconut water
4 cups baby spinach
¾ pear
½ apple
1 teaspoon green superfood
1-2 tablespoons lemon juice
1 cup of ice

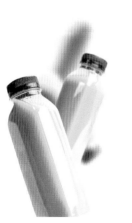

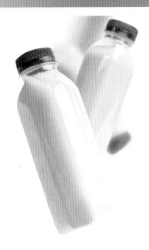

Dandelion and pineapple smoothie

1 ½ cups fresh pineapple
2 cups dandelion greens
2 cups baby spinach
1 ½ cups coconut water
Add all of the ingredients to the
blender except the coconut water.
Whisk in the coconut water before
serving.

Apple romaine smoothie

1 head of romaine lettuce
1 granny smith apple
½ lemon
Add all of the ingredients to the
blender

Sweet banana smoothie

1 cup unsweetened almond milk
1 cup of baby spinach
1 ½ frozen bananas
2 tablespoons almond butter
4 tablespoons organic plant based
protein
1 cup of ice

Peaches and green smoothie

1 ¾ cups unsweetened almond milk
2 cups baby spinach
1 tablespoon green superfood
½ frozen banana
2 cups peach slices
1 teaspoon spirulina
4 tablespoons organic plant based
protein

Watermelon blueberry smoothie

3 tablespoons chopped basil
1 ½ cup blueberries
2 pinches cayenne pepper
½ lime
5 cups diced watermelon
Add all ingredients to a blender

Apple and green smoothie

4 cups kale
1 apple
1 large cucumber
¼ lemon
Add all ingredients to a blender

Green smoothie

1 ½ cups unsweetened coconut milk
2 cups spinach
1 frozen banana
1 tablespoon spirulina
2 tablespoons chia seeds
1 tablespoon organic hemp seed
I cup ice

Dandelion smoothie

1 ½ cups unsweetened coconut milk
½ cup dandelion greens
2 cups baby spinach
1 frozen banana
½ kiwi fruit
1 tablespoon organic hemp seed
1 cup ice

Blueberries and almond smoothie

2 cups unsweetened almond milk
1 cup baby spinach
1 teaspoon spirulina
2 cups frozen blueberries
3 tablespoons almond butter
2 tablespoons chia seeds

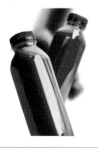

IN BRIEF

The consumption of vegetables is far more important than focussing on how they are prepared.

The food preparation method will determine how much you benefit from what you are eating.

Nutrients can be 'washed out' during cooking processes that involve water.

The raw food approach means that the body is not dealing with toxic residue as all food is consumed in its raw state.

The raw food diet is not suited to everyone. It is important that you gain the nutrients from food by preparing them in a way that makes them appetising.

It may be beneficial to consider raw consumption of certain foods and steaming others lightly which will increase your nutrient uptake.

The blending of raw fruit and vegetables together will increase nutrient intake and may make the blended approach more palatable.

Use of organic produce is always best.

Sugar - Possibly cancers best friend

Sugar is a fuel that all cells require and cancer cells are no different. By ingesting sugar, the pancreas produces insulin which is a hormone that helps to convert sugar in to energy for the body's cells.

Whilst it would be impossible to cut all sugar out of your diet, reducing and limiting processed sugar intake is needed to ensure cancer cells are not being fed. When we discuss the dangers of consuming sugar, we are referring to refined sugar which differs greatly to natural sugar.

Foods with natural sugar have an essential role in the diet of any individual trying to prevent cancer and especially for those fighting the disease. Refined sugar however, refers to sugars that have undergone an extraction and purification process so that they can easily be added to foods. When we look at sugar and cancer during this section, it is important to remember that we are referring to refined sugar and not natural sugar.

There are at least five reasons that cancer and sugar are possibly 'best friends.'

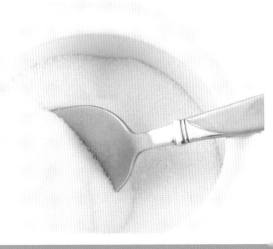

Affinity

Cancer cells possibly love sugar! That is why refined carbohydrates like white sugar, white flour, high fructose corn syrup (HFCS) and soft drinks are extremely dangerous for anyone trying to prevent or reverse cancer. Sugar essentially feeds tumours and encourages cancer growth. Cancer cells uptake sugar at an alarming rate in comparison to healthy cells. In fact, that is the basis of PET (positron emission tomography) scans used by the medical world to detect cancer growth. PET scans use radioactively labelled glucose to detect sugar-hungry tumour cells. When patients drink the sugar water, it gets preferentially taken up into the cancer cells and they light up. The 1931 Nobel laureate in medicine, German Otto Warburg, discovered that cancer cells have a fundamentally different energy metabolism compared to healthy cells. He found that malignant tumours exhibit increased glycolysis - a process whereby glucose is used as a fuel by cancer, compared with normal cells.

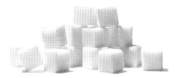

Acidity

Cancer cells thrive in an acidic environment and sugar is known to be highly acidic. With a pH of about 6.4, it is 10 times more acidic than the ideal alkaline pH of blood at approximately 7.4.

Immunity

Sugar suppresses a key immune response known as phagocytosis. This can be described as the Pac-Man effect of the immune system which is the ingestion of bacteria or other material. Consuming approximately 10 teaspoons of sugar can cause about a 50% reduction in phagocytosis. If you consider the sugar in your cereal, the sugar added to your morning coffee or tea, the sugar in cold beverages such as lemonade, and of course sugary snacks and desserts, you can see how easy it is to suppress your immune systems significantly. Not only the amount of sugar, but also the frequency of ingesting sugar is relevant to immune function. In one study, research subjects were found to have over a 30% decrease in phagocytosis one hour after ingesting a moderate amount of sugar. A couple of hours later, the immune system was suppressed by over 40%. Following from this, the immune system takes time to recover.

Activity

In most people, when sugar in any form is consumed the pancreas releases insulin. Breast tissue, for example, contains insulin receptors and insulin is a powerful stimulant of cell growth. One group of Australian researchers concluded that high levels of insulin and insulin-like growth factor (IGF) may actually be a significant factor in the development of cancers of the breast, prostate, endometrium and pancreas. Leading studies conducted in many countries in Europe, North America and Asia concluded that sugar intake is a strong risk factor contributing to higher breast cancer rates, particularly in older women.

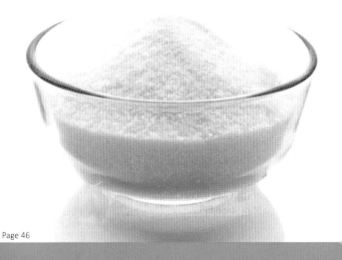

Obesity

Sugar ingestion seriously contributes to obesity, which may lead to the development of cancer. Obesity also negatively affects survival rates. More than 100,000 cases of cancer each year are caused by excess body fat, according to the American Institute for Cancer Research. These include oesophageal, pancreatic, kidney, gallbladder, breast and colorectal cancer.

Sugar Substitutes

Although sugar intake is not recommended, please do not take this to mean that sugar substitutes are a good alternative. Sweeteners containing aspartame, saccharin or sucralose have been shown to contribute to bladder cancer, lymphoma and leukaemia when used frequently according to the National Institute of Environmental Health Sciences.

Suggestions of better sugar substitutes are stevia (an all-natural herb from South America), barley malt, rice syrup, and palm sugar. Even high-glycaemic sweeteners, evaporated cane juice, molasses, honey and pure maple syrup are nutritionally superior to refined table sugar and you can avoid sugar spiking if you consume them in the presence of high fibre foods like ground flaxseeds.

IN BRIEF

Cancer cells thrive off refined sugar. It is known to feed tumours and encourage cancer growth.

Cancer cells uptake refined sugar approximately 10 times the rate of healthy cells.

Cancer cells thrive in an acidic environment – refined sugar is highly acidic.

Refined sugar supresses a key immune response called phagocytosis.

Refined sugar intake contributes to obesity, which has been suggested to be a cause of cancer.

Artificial sweeteners also come with risks so do not assume that using these as a substitute is a better option.

Insulin Potentiation Therapy (IPT) is an alternative cancer option that has almost none of the side effects such as nausea, hair loss and liver damage that potentially come from standard chemotherapy. Therefore it is an alternative option for those who chose chemotherapy as their chosen path as it allows this to be administered in a less damaging way.

This approach features an innovative low-dose chemotherapy protocol that uses 75-90% less chemotherapy than the traditional treatment to destroy cancer cells.

This is effective because cancer cells are known to have over 20 times more insulin sensitive receptors than normal healthy cells.

Cancer cells need glucose and this is one of the main sources of fuel that they use. As a result of this, cancer cells have approximately 20 times more insulin receptors on their surface than normal cells which enable the cells to absorb insulin when it is released by the pancreas following a meal. It is this insulin that is responsible for the delivery of glucose from the bloodstream, across cell membranes and into the cells.

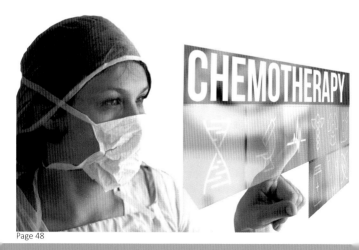

HOW DOES INSULIN WORK?

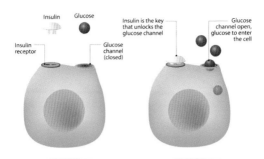

It is thought that slow growing cancer cells are less receptive to chemotherapy than fast growing cancer cells. Therefore to ensure that chemotherapy targets all cancer cells effectively, they must be fast growing and to push this process, a high glucose high insulin mix can be administered. Due to the abundance of insulin receptors on the surface of cancer cells, they have greater opportunity to take this glucose resource over normal cells. As a result, the fast growing cancer cells are more vulnerable to the administration of chemotherapy.

IPT involves the administration of insulin which triggers a drop in blood sugar in the body. This causes cancer cells to enter an emergency state and their membranes are open to enable them to obtain the sugar that they desperately need. Healthy cells however, shift to fat metabolism in this situation.

At this point a low dose of chemotherapy is administered followed quickly by sugar (glucose) which means that the cancer cells take in all of the chemotherapy in a desperate attempt to obtain the glucose they thrive off. It is believed that this method ensures that the cancer cells are targeted and due to the low dose of chemotherapy, there is little left to cause damage to healthy cells.

This differs greatly from the conventional chemotherapy

approach where potentially large doses of chemotherapy are administered and insulin is not used to open up the cancer cells. The result of this is that healthy cells are damaged in the process and the immune system is depleted further causing unpleasant side effects.

The process of Insulin Potentiation Therapy simply takes advantage of the highly active insulin receptors that cancer cells have. The word potentiation means that one substance (insulin) enhances the effectiveness of another substance (chemotherapy) and as a result, fewer drugs are required.

IPT is a consideration for those looking to incorporate chemotherapy into their treatment plan. It is well known that chemotherapy treatment comes with side effects and will damage healthy cells. IPT enables delivery of chemotherapeutic drugs at a low dose in conjunction with insulin to ensure that the treatment is targeted at cancer cells only. The result of this is reduced risk of side effects and a more effective treatment targeting the cells that you want to rid your body of.

IN BRIEF

Insulin Potentiation Therapy involves the use of insulin with low dose chemotherapy.

It ensures that side effects are reduced as the chemotherapy targets only the cancer cells.

Cancer cells thrive off sugar and for this reason, have approximately 20 times more insulin receptors on their surface than normal cells.

Insulin produced in the body delivers glucose (sugar) across cell membranes and into the cells to be used.

Insulin administration causes a drop in blood sugar and cancer cells open their membranes to enable them to obtain sugar resources.

Low dose chemotherapy is delivered followed by glucose which encourages the cancer cells to take on the chemotherapy in an attempt to obtain sugar.

The cancer cells are targeted leaving the healthy, non-sugar dependant cells intact.

It is the damage to healthy cells that is the root cause of chemotherapy side effects. Therefore these are prevented.

Fruits and vegetables are the best sources of vitamin C and foods such as citrus fruits, tomatoes, peppers, kiwifruit and strawberries are all rich in this essential vitamin. It is fortunate that some of the best sources of vitamin C are usually consumed in their raw state which prevents any loss of nutrition during the cooking process. By simply increasing your oral intake of vitamin C, you will gain the benefit of this powerful anti-oxidant which will empower your immune system and help you in the fight against cancer

Vitamin C is required for the growth, development and repair of all tissues in the body. It is also involved in many body functions including the formation of collagen, absorption of iron, the immune system, wound healing and the maintenance of cartilage, bones and teeth.

Oral vitamin C is a known antioxidant that limits the damaging effects of free radicals. It can therefore help to prevent or delay the development of certain cancers alongside other diseases.

Remember that empowerment of the immune system is paramount.

Vitamin C is just one of those components that the immune system needs on a regular daily basis to enable it to function to its full potential. The importance of vitamin C is highlighted when we consider that many people, particularly sea men lost their lives to a disease called scurvy. It was then discovered that scurvy was not actually a disease and was simply caused by a deficiency of vitamin C which is of course, easily prevented.

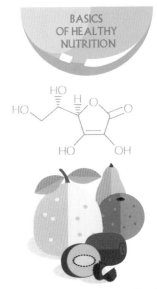

BASICS OF HEALTHY NUTRITION

Vitamin C
Ascorbic acid
is a naturally occurring organic compound with antioxidant properties.

TOP
10
VITAMIN C
CONTENTS

per 100 g product

Rosehip fruit	650 mg
Red sweet pepper	250 mg
Sea buckthorn	200 mg
Blackcurrant	181 mg
Kiwi	180 mg
Parsley leaves	150 mg
Brussels sprouts	100 mg
Lichee	71,5 mg
Rowanberry	70 mg
Cauliflower	70 mg
Pomelo	61 mg
Papaya	60,9 mg
Scotch kale	60 mg
Strawberry	60 mg
Spinach	55 mg
Lemon	53 mg
Kohlrabi cabbage	50 mg
White cabbage	45 mg
Orange	45 mg
Grapefruit	31,2 mg
Lemon	30 mg
Mango	28 mg
Mandarin	26,7 mg

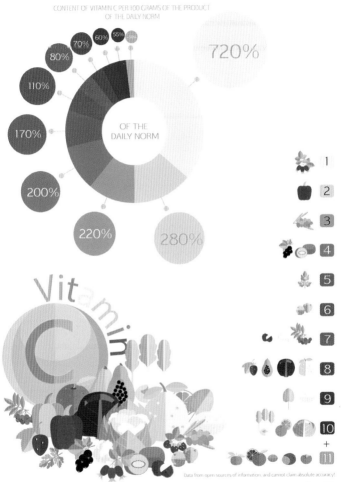

CONTENT OF VITAMIN C PER 100 GRAMS OF THE PRODUCT
OF THE DAILY NORM

720%

60% 55% 50%

70%

80%

110%

170%

OF THE
DAILY NORM

200%

220%   280%

Data from open sources of information and cannot claim absolute accuracy!

Oral Vitamin C - A Powerful Antioxidant

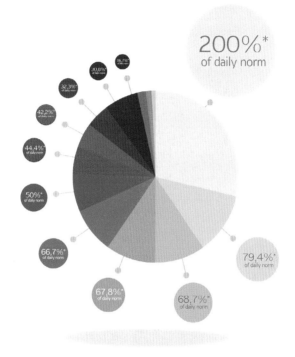

200%*
of daily norm

36,7%*
of daily norm

30,8%*
of daily norm

32,3%*
of daily norm

42,2%*
of daily norm

44,4%*
of daily norm

50%*
of daily norm

66,7%*
of daily norm

67,8%*
of daily norm

68,7%*
of daily norm

79,4%*
of daily norm

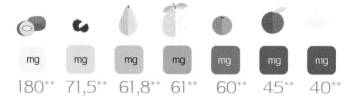

mg	mg	mg	mg	mg	mg	mg
180**	71,5**	61,8**	61**	60**	45**	40**

**Contents per 100 grams of product in milligrams.

Oral Vitamin C - A Powerful Antioxidant

- Kiwi
- Lichee
- Papaya
- Pomelo
- Orange
- Grapefruit
- Lemon
- Tangerine
- Lime
- Mango
- Persimmon

- Cherry
  Pineapple
  Apple
  Pomegranate
  Apricot
  Avocado
  Banana
  Plum
- Cherries
  Grapes
  Watermelon
  Peach
- Pear
  Figs

IN BRIEF

Oral vitamin C is just one component that the body needs on a regular daily basis to enable it to function to its full potential.

Oral vitamin C is a powerful antioxidant that limits the damaging effects of free radicals.

It can assist in the prevention and delay in development of certain cancers.

Oral vitamin C is found in many fruits and vegetable.

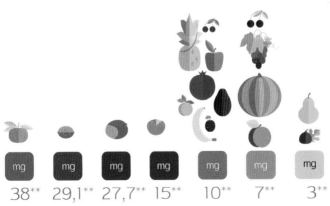

mg	mg	mg	mg	mg	mg	mg
38**	29,1**	27,7**	15**	10**	7**	3**

Data from open sources of information, and cannot claim absolute accuracy!

As a result of its known benefits, it is common sense to view vitamin C as a useful source to help to prevent and help to fight cancer. Further to dietary intake of vitamin C, there is now great interest in the use of high dose vitamin C as an effective cancer treatment. Throughout this section we will make reference to the intravenous administration of vitamin C. This refers to how this option is administered in to the body and in this instance; it is by injection of vitamin C into a vein. This procedure is carried out only by professional healthcare practitioners and always within a clinical setting.

Research shows that vitamin C is selectively cytotoxic to cancer cells when administered intravenously in high doses and also has a number of heart and cardiovascular benefits. When given intravenously at high doses, vitamin C produces a pro-oxidant effect, thereby generating hydrogen peroxide which ultimately helps with the destruction of cancer cells. Normal tissues are not harmed by the high levels of hydrogen peroxide generated because healthy

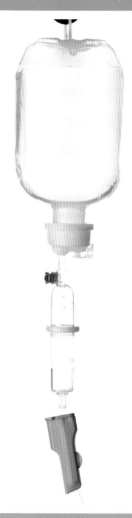

cells have several ways of effectively removing it This prevents build up to toxic levels and cancer cells lack this ability.

In order for vitamin C to effectively help to destroy cancer cells, a very high concentration of vitamin C is needed in your blood and the only way to obtain these levels is through IV administration. By bypassing the digestive tract, IV administration results in blood levels up to 500 times higher than the levels that can be achieved through the oral route.

The mechanism behind vitamin C's ability to selectively target cancer cells has to do with the generation of hydrogen peroxide which is ultimately what helps to kill the cancer cells. Cancer cells are much more prone to damage and death from a high amount of hydrogen peroxide which explains why high levels of vitamin C do not affect normal tissue but can damage tumour tissue. Healthy cells have several ways of effectively removing hydrogen peroxide which therefore prevents a toxic build up and tumour cells are unable to do this.

One of the primary pathways of hydrogen peroxide removal is the enzyme catalase, and it has been found that cells with reduced catalase activity are indeed more prone to die when exposed to high amounts of IV vitamin C.

This provides a hint at which cancers are likely the best candidates for high-dose IV vitamin C therapy. Tumours with low catalase levels are likely to be the most responsive, whereas tumours with high catalase levels would be the least responsive. Treatment with high-dose vitamin C has been proven to slow the growth of prostate, pancreatic, liver, colon, malignant mesothelioma, neuroblastoma and other types of cancer cells.

IV vitamin C is also known to act as an anti-inflammatory. As a general rule, chronic inflammation is a hallmark of cancer and it has been noted that IV vitamin C treatment helps lower pro-inflammatory cytokines and C-reactive protein which are two inflammatory markers. This reduction directly correlates with a reduction in tumour size. A reduction in inflammation around tumour sites will in turn, reduce any symptoms caused by pressure on surrounding structures within the body. Therefore the anti-inflammatory properties are twofold.

IV vitamin C can also help to lower the risk of metastasis which is the spread of the disease from the original site. This was shown in a study conducted by the Riordan Clinic, the successor to Linus Pauling and his valuable work on IV vitamin C. A positive response was noted in over 70% of patients. There is likely no clinic in the world with as much experience with IV vitamin C as the Riordan Clinic. Riordan carried out a 15-year-long research project called RECNAC (cancer spelled backwards), which showed IV vitamin C was selectively cytotoxic against cancer cells.

Other research conducted by scientists at the Lewis Cantley of Weill Cornel Medicine in New York found high doses of IV vitamin C helps kill and eliminate colorectal cancer cells with certain genetic mutations.

Given in high doses, IV vitamin C acts as a pro-oxidant and therefore oxidises tissues which is exactly what chemotherapy does. The high plasma concentrations of IV vitamin C that comes from IV administration lead to the generation of free radicals causing the IV vitamin C to act as a pro-oxidant. Human studies also show IV vitamin C can help improve symptoms associated with cancer and cancer treatment, such as fatigue, nausea, vomiting, pain and loss of appetite, and improve overall quality of life.

While the evidence strongly supports the use of IV vitamin C in high doses for infections, inflammation and even cancer, administering IV vitamin C is not for the novice. It is strongly recommended that an experienced practitioner is consulted if selecting IV vitamin C therapy. This will ensure that is carried out in a safe manner and all necessary checks are carried out prior to undergoing the therapy.

Intravenous Vitamin C (A Powerful Pro-oxidant)

It is essential that any practitioner administering IV vitamin C checks your glucose-6-phosphate dehydrogenase (G6PD). G6PD is an enzyme that red blood cells need to maintain membrane integrity. High-dose IV vitamin C is actually a strong pro-oxidant, and giving a pro-oxidant to a G6PD-deficient individual can cause haemolysis (rupturing) of their red blood cells. This deficiency is rare but is important to mention for those considering this route.

There are places across the UK that will carry out the G6PD blood test. In our experience and from the research we carried out; it is significantly cheaper to have IV vitamin C therapy abroad.

Therefore, the importance of IV vitamin C is something to give consideration to, alongside the other approaches in this guide when deciding on your own individual journey. High dose IV vitamin C is not for everyone but by providing the background and benefits to this treatment, informed choices can then be made.

IN BRIEF

Administered in high doses intravenously, vitamin C becomes a pro-oxidant.

High doses of vitamin C can be given intravenously and can damage tumour tissue while leaving healthy tissue intact.

Vitamin C becomes a pro-oxidant when given in high doses.

A G6PD test is required before undergoing high dose IV vitamin C therapy.

Please consult a health care professional.

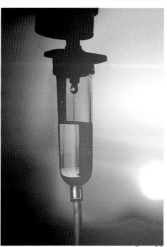

Lemons

Lemons have been proven to have strong anti-cancer properties in addition to the many other useful qualities of this fruit. Lemons have an exceptionally solid impact on cysts and tumours by annihilating the cancer-causing cells of more than 10 types of cancers. Lemons also help to prevent the spread of cancer-causing cells.

In addition to the vitamin C found in lemon juice, the peel of the fruit can be of benefit in the elimination of toxins from the body. Due to the versatility of lemons, it is easy enough to ensure that these can be added in to your daily diet. Very simply squeezing a lemon into the water you drink throughout the day will ensure you are benefiting from the power of this fruit.

In the event that you include baking soda with lemon it will act as a more superior treatment on the grounds that in this way, the pH estimation

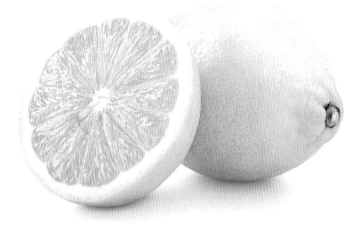

of the body will be standardized. By including baking soda with lemons you will effectively help to diminish the acidity of the body. The diseased cells in the body will struggle to develop in an alkaline domain.

Lemons have a strong anticancer effect. It has been proven that they help to destroy the malignant cells of more than 10 types of cancer, including colon, breast, prostate, lung and pancreas. When the baking soda is added to the lemon, the effect is even greater because it completely changes the pH levels of the body.

Try combining the following to make a drink to reduce acidity in the body. This is best consumed on an empty stomach and can be consumed three times a day.

1 teaspoon of baking soda

200mls. lemon juice

You can dilute the mixture with some purified water

What is really important is that this drink does not have the side effects typical of conventional cancer treatments. Therefore it is worth considering as an addition to your treatment choices.

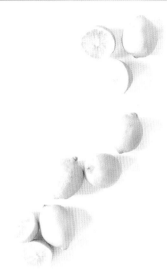

IN BRIEF

Lemons are a valuable source of vitamin C.

Lemons are an inexpensive option and are easily obtained.

Lemons have strong anti-cancer properties.

It has been found that lemons help to to prevent the spread of cancer-causing cells.

Try to purchase wax free organic lemons where possible.

The health benefits of honey are well documented. However, the naturally occurring active agent which is thought to support good health is destroyed when exposed to heat and light. Manuka honey contains an additional naturally occurring active ingredient which sets it apart from other types of honey. This additional component is stable and doesn't lose potency when it is diluted or exposed to heat and light.

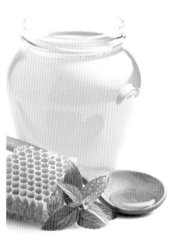

This special quality is known as UMF which stands for Unique Manuka Factor. This is a quality trademark and grading system that appraises the natural markers found in Manuka honey and gives the assurance of quality and purity. UMF 16+ is considered to be superior high grade Manuka honey whilst literature suggests that anything above UMF 10 will have the potency required to deliver the health benefits of this special honey.

Manuka honey is considered to be nature's version of liquid gold and has many additional health benefits in comparison to other types of honey. Manuka honey is made by bees that pollinate the Manuka flowers that grow almost exclusively in the East Cape region of New Zealand. It is this honey's exclusivity alongside its medicinal properties that makes it expensive.

The health benefits of Manuka honey are vast. This honey has antiviral and antibacterial properties and dozens of species of bacteria appear to be susceptible to Manuka honey, including MRSA and Clostridium difficile which spread within healthcare settings and are difficult to treat. There are no known reports of microbial resistance to Manuka honey which suggests that it may be a successful option against resistant organisms and prolonged wound infections that cannot be treated with antibiotic therapy.

Manuka honey can be used topically to alleviate skin complaints by reducing inflammation and irritation in conditions like eczema and acne. It is widely used for wound healing from burns and bacterial skin infections to infected ulcers on the skin.

Use of Manuka honey orally will benefit the digestive system and ease symptoms of throat infections and irritable bowel disease.

Manuka honey is loaded with antioxidants which are known to benefit our health at the same time as boosting our energy levels. It is superior in mineral content and provides the body with calcium, phosphorous, iron, zinc, copper, sodium, potassium, magnesium and manganese in varied amounts. Those who use Manuka honey as part of their daily routine report increased resistance to illness and disease.

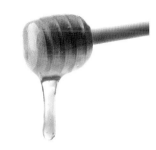

The immune reactions in the body involve the signalling proteins called cytokines. These are what trigger the defence mechanisms in the body and push the fight against pathogens and diseases. It has been found that Manuka honey has the ability to stimulate and increase the production of cytokines which in turn is how it boosts the immune system and protects against potential infections and diseases.

Introducing Manuka honey into your daily diet is an easy way to boost your immune system. Remember to shop wisely and look for the important UMF rating before you purchase to ensure that the honey is of high quality and will provide you with the full health benefits. Seek Manuka honey with UMF 10+ or if possible, UMF 16+.

DRINKS | CEREALS & BEANS | NUTS | FRUITS & BERRIES | VEGETABLES | SPICES & HERBS | MEAT & POULTRY | DAIRY & EGGS | FISH | SEAFOOD | OILS | DESSERTS

FOOD COLLECTION
infographics

HONEY

VITAMINS
PER 100 g
MINERALS

0.5 mg — C — Ascorbic Acid

0.121 mg — B3 — Niacin

0.068 mg — B5 — Pantothenic Acid

0.038 mg — B2 — Riboflavin

0.024 mg — B6 — Pyridoxine

0.01 mg — B1 — Thiamine

2 µg — B9 — Folic Acid

52 mg — K — Potassium

6 mg — Ca — Calcium

4 mg — P — Phosphorus

4 mg — Na — Sodium

2 mg — Mg — Magnesium

0.8 mg — Se — Selenium

0.42 mg — Fe — Iron

Nutritional value per 100 g

PROTEINS	LIPIDS	CARBOHYDRATES	WATER
0.3 g	0 g	82.4 g	17.1 g

Strengthens the immune system, has antibacterial & antifungal effect

ENERGY

Contains antioxidants, prevents heart disease, can help lower blood pressure

Reduces gastrointestinal disorders, possesses large amount of friendly bacteria

304 kcal

Promotes burn & wound healing

As a guide, consume 1-2 tablespoons of raw Manuka honey as part of your daily routine. Alternatively, spread on toast or drizzle over fruit if you struggle to consume the honey on its own as you will still benefit from the medicinal properties it offers.

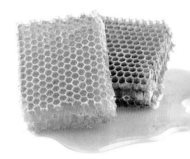

IN BRIEF

Manuka honey is made by bees from the nectar of the Manuka bush found in New Zealand.

Manuka honey is seen as the gold standard honey with regards to health benefits and medicinal properties.

It is graded by the Unique Manuka Factor (UMF) – the higher the number, the greater the action of the honey.

Seek Manuka honey with UMF 10+ to ensure you are gaining the true benefits or opt for UMF 16+ for superior grade Manuka honey if possible.

Manuka honey is known to have antiviral and antibacterial properties.

It can be used orally or topically depending on the ailment it is being used for.

Manuka honey stimulates the production of cytokines which is how it boosts the immune system and protects against potential infections and diseases.

As a guide, incorporate 1-2 tablespoons of Manuka honey into your daily diet to benefit from its medicinal properties.

The apricot kernel is the soft part found inside the seed of the apricot. It is an excellent source of iron, potassium and phosphorous and is the best source of amygdalin or laetrile as it is often known as.

There are two types of apricot kernels – bitter and sweet. It is the bitter kernel that is known for its therapeutic values. Laetrile is believed to fight cancer by targeting and helping to kill cancer cells whilst building the immune system to help prevent recurrence. However, there is much controversy surrounding the use of laetrile which was banned by the Food and Drug Administration (FDA) in the 1980's and has practically disappeared within the mainstream medical community.

Laetrile is a partly synthetic form of the natural product amygdalin. Amygdalin is a plant substance found in raw nuts and the pips of many fruits – particularly apricot kernels or pips. Some consider laetrile to be vitamin B17 although this term maybe inaccurate. The term vitamin B17 was used to insinuate that this was a dietary supplement for retail purposes. We will use this term as it is well known

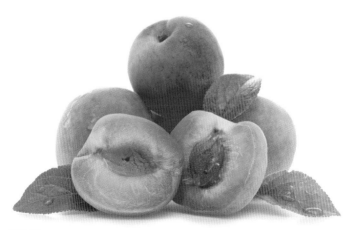

and is often used alongside laetrile and amygdalin.

Healthy cells contain the enzyme rhodanese which protects the cells by neutralising the benzaldehyde and cyanide in B17 and converts them into useful compounds. Cancer cells do not have rhodanese. Instead they have an enzyme called beta-glucosidase which unlocks the benzaldehyde and cyanide from the glucose to create a poison which helps to kill the cancer cells. The selective killing effects of vitamin B17 on mutated cells is called apoptosis which is a mechanism of 'programmed cell death' and destroys cancer cells readily, whilst leaving health cells alone.

In a study by the Department of Physiology at Kyung Hee University in South Korea, amygdalin extract was combined with cancerous human prostate cells. The extract helped significantly induce apoptosis in the prostate cancer cells. The researchers concluded that amygdalin may offer a valuable, natural option for prostate cancer. Other animal studies show that vitamin B17 amygdalin is effective at killing cancerous bladder and brain cells under certain conditions, especially when combined with other antibody-enzyme complexes.

Vitamin B17 contains special properties that help to slow down the spread of illness throughout the body by killing harmful cells, but the exact way that vitamin B17 does this is not fully understood.

A study published in the International Journal of Radiation and Biology found that vitamin B17 amygdalin stimulated the immune system by causing a statistically significant increase in the ability of a patient's white blood cells to attack harmful cells. One theory of vitamin B17's effects suggests that transformation of normal cells into dangerous cells that can cause disease is normally prevented by beneficial enzymes produced within the pancreas. So vitamin B17 may help increase the production of pancreatic enzymes that destroy harmful properties within the body.

Vitamin B17 is also thought to help the body experience enhanced detoxification effects by supporting liver function. This boosts immune function by eliminating harmful toxins, malignant cells and other potentially damaging substances before they cause illness or serious chronic diseases. Another explanation of vitamin B17 mechanisms is that when vitamin B17 releases cyanide, it increases the acid content of tumours and helps with the destruction of harmful cells within the tumours which in turn arrests their growth.

Because the evidence available does not give clear assurance of the safety of this therapy, it is recommended that vitamin B17 is best obtained from natural food sources as opposed to high doses of synthetic supplements. While it is common sense that this will provide a much lower dose, it is deemed to be the safest form of obtaining vitamin B17 and poses less risk than other options.

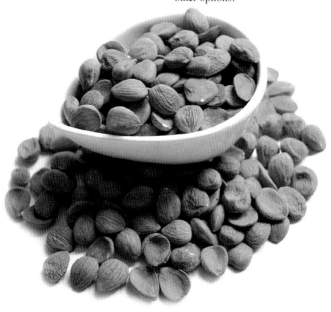

As mentioned previously, the most common source of vitamin B17 is apricot kernels and bitter almonds. However, almost all seeds and kernels from various types of fruits such as apple seeds and pear seeds contain vitamin B17. Beans and certain whole grains also contain vitamin B17.

The exact amount of vitamin B17 within foods is not well-known, and levels are thought to vary widely within a food depending on where it's grown, the quality of the soil and how fresh it is.

Vitamin B17 is not a new phenomenon and for those who are unsure as to whether it is a safe option, it is important to understand the history behind it and its medicinal properties. Bitter almonds are known as being a source of vitamin B17 and have been used as a traditional remedy for thousands of years by ancient Egyptians, Chinese and Pueblo Indians. The compounds in vitamin B17 were discovered in the early 1800's when a chemist realized that distilling the water from bitter almonds released hydrocyanic acid and this could be purified to form amygdalin, the active ingredient of vitamin B17.

Vitamin B17 in the form of laetrile was first used as a cancer treatment in Russia back in the mid-1800s and then spread to the United States in the early 1900's. By the 1970s, laetrile gained popularity as an anti-cancer agent, with more than 70,000 individuals in the U.S. alone using vitamin B17 laetrile to help fight cancer.

At this time, there is no established recommended daily value of vitamin B17 However, many doctors specialising in cancer treatment use vitamin B17 (or laetrile) in relatively high doses without patients commonly experiencing side effects.

Currently, the administration, schedules and the duration of taking vitamin B17 vary widely depending on the patient's specific condition and the practitioner prescribing it. Part of the trouble determining exactly how and how much vitamin B17 can be beneficial is that much of the research using vitamin B17 took place in the 1970s and '80s but was discontinued since the ban in the 1980s.

A popular way to consume vitamin B17 is eating apricot kernels. In the

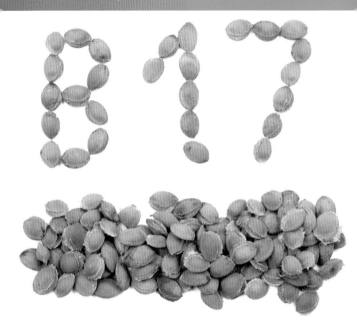

middle of an apricot, or other fruit seeds like a peach pit or apple seed, there is a hard shell that can be broken into. Once broken, a small seed/kernel in the middle is found that looks something like a small almond — this is the part of the fruit that's naturally high in vitamin B17.

Experts usually recommend eating 25–40 kernels per day for disease prevention or about 16 kernels and

upwards for maintenance. It is important to note that a starting dose of 1 per day can be taken and then intake must be increased gradually. Therefore it may take a few weeks to build up to a dose of 25-40 per day.

The common sense approach to vitamin B17 therapy if you consider this to be a suitable option would be to naturally increase your intake of vitamin B17 through food sources like those we have mentioned. Obtaining your nutrients from whole foods is the best approach as this eliminates any possible concerns regarding synthetic fillers or toxins alongside the potential for overdosing that come with using questionable extracts and supplements.

To enable you to make an informed decision regarding vitamin B17, it is essential that you are aware of the possibility of experiencing side effects from this therapy. Other therapies discussed in this guide do not have known side effects attached to them but vitamin B17 is the exception and it is important that you have an awareness of these.

While we acknowledge that vitamin B17 is not for everyone dealing with a cancer diagnosis, it has an importance in the world of alternative approaches and can therefore not be ignored. Whilst it is recognised that research is limited, by presenting you with the available current information you will be forearmed to decide whether this is an approach that will be suited to you.

IN BRIEF

Apricot kernels are a rich source of laetrile (B17)

Laetrile is known to target and help to kill cancer cells whilst building the immune system.

Vitamin B17 is also thought to help the body experience enhanced detoxification effects by supporting liver function.

The purchase of vitamin B17 laetrile supplements is illegal and almost impossible to obtain.

A popular, effective way of ingesting vitamin B17 is by eating apricot kernels which is completely natural and legal.

Therapeutic doses are unknown as much research was carried out in the 1970's and 80's and is no longer permitted.

Apricot kernels must be slowly introduced into your system.

Curcumin is the yellow pigment in the spice turmeric. Studies have shown that this element of turmeric has anticancer effects on cancerous cells within the body. The anticancer effects of curcumin extend beyond its ability to potentially prevent DNA mutations. It also appears to help regulate programmed cell death.

Our cells are pre-programmed to die naturally to make way for fresh cells in a process known as apoptosis. In a sense, your body is rebuilding itself every few months with the materials you provide through your diet. Some cells however, overstay their welcome such as cancer cells. By somehow disabling their own suicide mechanism, they do not die when they are supposed to and they continue to thrive and divide. This results in the development of tumours which can potentially spread throughout the body.

So what impact does curcumin have on this process?

Curcumin appears to have the ability to re-programme the self-destruct

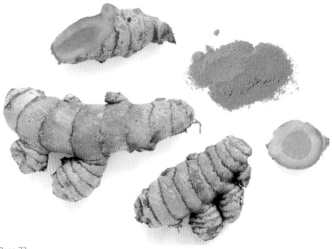

The anticancer properties of the spice curcumin

mechanism back into cancer cells. All cells contain so called death receptors that trigger the self-destruction sequence but cancer cells can disable their own death receptors. Curcumin however appears to be able to reactivate them. It can also help to kill cancer cells directly by activating the execution enzymes called caspases inside cancer cells that destroy them from within by chopping up their proteins. Unlike most chemotherapy drugs, which cancer cells over time can develop resistance to, curcumin affects several mechanisms of cell death simultaneously which in turn makes it harder for cancer cells to avoid destruction. Curcumin has been found to be effective against a variety of cancer cells invitro including those of the breast, blood, colon, brain, kidney, liver, lungs and skin. For reasons not understood, curcumin seems to leave non-cancerous cells alone.

Pancreatic cancer is among the most aggressive forms of cancer and untreated and most patients may potentially die from this. Unfortunately only a small percentage of patients appear to respond to chemotherapy with the majority of these suffering severe side effects. Curcumin appears to be able to help to reverse pre-cancerous changes in colon cancer and has been shown in studies, to be effective against lung cancer cells. Similar results were obtained against pancreatic cancerous cells.

So why not try using curcumin to treat patients with pancreatic cancer? In a study funded by the National Cancer Institute and performed at the MD Anderson Cancer Centre, patients with advanced pancreatic cancer were given large doses of curcumin. Out of over 20 of the patients involved in the study, the researchers were able to evaluate that 2 responded positively to the treatment. One patient had over 70% reduction in his tumour size although eventually, a curcumin resistant tumour developed in its place. The remaining patients showed steady improvement over the course of 18 months. The only time when cancer markers were seen to increase was during a brief 3 week period when the curcumin therapy was halted. It may be that the tumours of only 2 out of over 21 participants responded, but it is important to remember that this is approximately the same as the response you would see from a chemotherapy regime. Zero adverse effects were reported by those involved in the study due to it being a natural spice.

Therefore, it is a common sense suggestion that pancreatic cancer patients take curcumin regardless of other routes they may chose. Given the tragic prognosis of this cancer, prevention is critical and until we know more, we must use all the available options to us.

Use of a natural spice with no side effects and can be purchased at low cost will empower your immune system.

IN BRIEF

Curcumin is known to have anticancer properties.

It also appears to have no harmful effect on healthy cells in the body.

It reactivates the death receptors in cancer cells that help to trigger the self-destruction sequence.

Curcumin is a natural spice that has no known side effects and aids empowerment of the immune system.

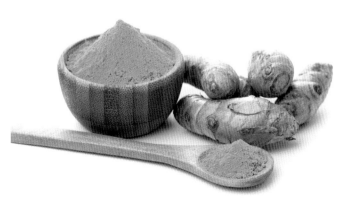

Selenium is a mineral found in the soil, which naturally appears in water and certain foods. Selenium is a potential cancer fighter as it is a known antioxidant and therefore has the ability to protect cells from damage.

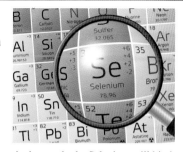

Research shows that increased levels of selenium lower the risk of cancer and are an important component in the fight against cancer. Garlic, onion, broccoli and wholegrains are on the National Cancer Institute's list of foods that can reduce the risk of developing cancer and these are foods rich in selenium.

Toxic chemicals surround us in the environment. One such chemical is mercury which is a biological toxin that can be lethal and can have a detrimental impact on the brain, kidneys and liver as it binds to fatty tissue with ease. Mercury competes with essential minerals and a deficiency in minerals allows a mercury accumulation in cells which in turn shuts down antioxidant systems. The mineral selenium is an effective detoxifying agent which is known to prevent high concentrations of mercury in the human body. Selenium will bind with toxins in the body and has the ability to neutralise harmful activity and when selenium and mercury bind, the new compound it forms is excreted as waste as it cannot be absorbed into the body. This has massive health benefits and therefore it is common sense that the presence of selenium is one of the most effective ways to remove any accumulated mercury from the body. We must ensure that we include a surplus of selenium to reduce mercury levels. Selenium is also known to be one of the best anti-inflammatory sources and can regulate the immune response and improve blood flow.

By increasing selenium levels, the natural antioxidant defence system of cells is enhanced. It has the ability to bind protective antioxidants to the areas of our DNA that require repair which reduces cancer growth and impacts on the ageing process. Selenium contributes to natural antioxidant pathways which serve to stimulate cell death in cancer cells. Therefore, whilst selenium is known to prevent cancer developing, it also has been shown to aid the slowing of cancer progression which contributes to cancer reversal.

As far back as the 1960's, research has identified that low blood levels of selenium may be associated with an increased risk of cancer. Through the years, scientists have built a persuasive case that a selenium rich diet may protect against cancer. What is even more exciting is that recent studies offer compelling evidence that selenium supplements may greatly reduce the risk of developing many different common cancers. Research shows that there is a strong link between low selenium levels and higher incidence of cancer occurrence.

The Willett study, headed by Dr Walter C Willet of Harvard was conducted at several research centres throughout the United States

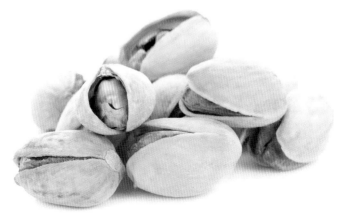

of America in 1973. Blood samples were collected from over 4000 men in 14 regions of the country. At the time of drawing the samples, none of the participants had any signs of cancer. Over the next 5 years, over 100 men from this group developed cancer. The blood samples from these men were analysed and compared against samples from over 200 healthy men who were matched for age and lifestyle except they had no signs of cancer. The study clearly demonstrated that the men with the lowest selenium blood levels were twice as likely to have developed cancer compared to those with the highest levels. The following year, Cornell University researchers compared the blood selenium levels of skin cancer patients to those who did not have cancer. Once again, they found that those with the lowest selenium levels were over 5 times more likely to develop skin cancer compared to those with higher levels.

So how much selenium is required?

Most people will obtain their recommended daily allowance of selenium from food. Brazil nuts, yellowfin tuna, pumpkin seeds, sardines and spinach are all foods rich in selenium. However, for the protection against cancer and to fight cancer once it has been detected, it is recommended that a supplement of around 200mcgs per day would be of great benefit. It is worth noting that selenium taken with vitamin E is favourable as they facilitate each other's absorption

IN BRIEF

Selenium has been shown to be essential in the fight against cancer.

It is a known detoxifying agent and prevents a build-up of mercury in the body.

It is an effective anti-inflammatory and has the ability to regulate the immune response.

Increased selenium levels enhance the natural antioxidant defence systems of cells.

Selenium can aid in the prevention of cancer and can also assist in the decelerating of cancer progression.

It is recommended that in addition to selenium obtained from diet, a therapeutic dose of around 200mcgs of selenium daily will be beneficial.

Take selenium with vitamin E for better absorption.

Black Seed

Black seeds are the seeds of the nigella sativa flowering plant which is commonly known as fennel flower. Black seeds and the oil pressed from them have been used in traditional medicine in certain cultures for centuries.

It is thought that black seed dates back as far as over 3000 years. The earliest record of its cultivation and use come from ancient Egypt. Black seed oil it is said was found in Egyptian Pharaoh Tutankhamun's tomb. In Arabic cultures, black cumin is known as Habbatul barakah, meaning the "seed of blessing." Many of black cumin's traditionally ascribed health benefits have been thoroughly confirmed in biomedical literature. In fact, since the early 1960's, there have been over 450 published, peer-reviewed studies referencing it.

Black seed oil has therapeutic benefits and when taken internally, it can assist with combatting disease. There is evidence to demonstrate that this oil can help to inhibit the growth of cancerous tumours in the colon, lungs, oesophagus and stomach based on a study conducted using rats. It was found that black seed oil has the ability to supress the proliferation of cancerous cells. Therefore the study concluded that black seed oil has the potential to prevent the development of cancerous tumours and in the early stages of cancer, could prevent the need for chemotherapy treatment.

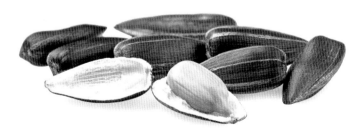

As proof that black seed oil is making headway as a remedy for cancer, in America the Food and Drug Administration (FDA) has granted two patents that involve this oil for the purpose of cancer treatment. The FDA has recognised the ability of black seed oil in empowering the immune system and helping to prevent the growth of cancerous cells. One of the interesting facts about black seed oil is that it isn't selective and appears to work on all cancer types.

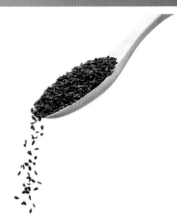

A recent study in America looked at black seed oil and pancreatic tumours and found that black seed destroyed pancreatic cancer cells at a rapid rate. It was also discovered that there was an increase in the growth rate of bone marrow cells by over 200% which proves its immune boosting properties. As well as being an excellent natural treatment, black seed oil can be used as a natural protector against the damage radiation and chemotherapy can cause to the immune system by protecting healthy tissue from oxidative stress.

In 2014, Saudi Arabian researchers conducted a study on the benefits of black seed oil for lung cancer patients. This research used human lung cancer cells and found that the use of black seed oil significantly reduced the number of living cancer cells present. In addition to this, it was evident that the greater the concentration of oil used had a direct correlation to the increased level of cell death observed. It was also noted that the black seed oil caused the cancer cells to shrink and lose their typical appearance.

Black seed oil can be easily purchased although there are some important considerations when selecting this product. It is essential to ensure that the oil purchased is organic and pure-pressed without chemical extraction. High quality black seed oil will contain no additives or diluting oils. This should be stored in light-protective and air-sealed glass.

The required dosage of black seed oil is difficult to state due to the limited available research conducted on humans. There are many suggestions related to this on the internet and from patient experience. On reviewing the suggestions available, it appears that one teaspoon of high quality black seed

oil seems to give therapeutic benefit if consumed 2-3 times per day. As a preventative measure, one teaspoon once per day seems to be the common dosage.

IN BRIEF

The history of black seed oil is well known and has been used safely history suggests, since the time of the Egyptian Pharaohs.

It is apparent that black seed oil is beneficial when used alone or in conjunction with conventional cancer treatments.

Black seed oil can help to supress the proliferation of cancerous cells in the body.

It is proven to help to reduce the side effects from radiation by preventing damage to healthy tissue.

Black seed oil helps to rebuild the immune system and helps to destroy cancer cells.

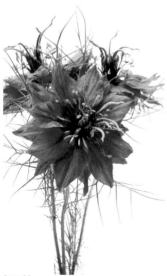

PH levels refer to a measure of alkalinity of water soluble substances and pH stands for 'potential of Hydrogen'. The pH balance of the body is essential for maintaining a healthy body and the ideal pH is slightly alkaline – which is between 7.30 and 7.45. The pH level of the body impacts all cells, tissues, glands, organs, and organ systems. Increasing your alkalinity to the ideal range will alleviate stress on your organ systems right down to individual cells which in turn, will assist your body to fight off illness and disease.

What is pH balance?

The potential for hydrogen (pH) balance of our body is measured on a scale of 0 to 14, 7 being neutral, less than 7 being acidic and greater than 7 being alkaline. The higher the hydrogen concentration, the more acidic a substance will become. The human body stays at a stable alkaline level of approximately 7.36 – significant shifts from this number can be life threatening. In fact, the body strives very hard to maintain this balance unless there are foreign viruses or cancerous cells attacking it. Modern medicine has suggested that what we ingest cannot significantly alter the acidity or the alkalinity of our bloodstream. The body has a complex system that makes sure the blood stays in its healthy, slightly alkaline range. If blood becomes too acidic or too alkaline, the body automatically corrects this on its own. Your blood may become slightly more acid or alkaline after eating certain foods – but it will stay within the healthy range without a special diet.

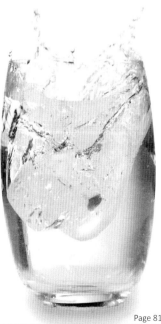

The Importance of pH to the body

While the modern diet has become more acidic than ever before, our bodies faithfully maintain their bloodstream's normal pH range.

So why should you be concerned?

Our bodies may naturally work to maintain a stable pH and in doing so, keep us healthy. However, if we don't give our bodies what they require to maintain this balance in a healthy fashion, we pay the price in other ways.

Our blood achieves the pH balance by using important minerals from our organs, glands, tissues and bones. Calcium in the form of phosphates and carbonates represents a large reservoir of base in our body. In response to an acid load such as the modern diet, these salts are released into the systemic circulation to bring the pH into homeostasis. It has been estimated that the quantity of calcium lost in the urine with the modern diet over time could be as high as almost half the skeletal mass of calcium over 20 years. Our kidneys are one of the main cleansing portals that help flush excess acid from our blood stream. The kidneys help regulate the acid/alkaline balance of the

bloodstream by eliminating solid acids, also known as fixed acids – especially sulphuric and uric acid – through urination. If acid wastes cannot be eliminated, they get re-absorbed, re-filtered through the liver, and released into circulation, which facilitates free radicals and various bacteria. This acid waste is caused by overly acidic food, like processed snacks, sugar, pasteurized dairy, and meat.

One can of cola contains enough phosphoric acid to dramatically change our pH. The pH of the cola is between 2.8 and 3.2, but the kidneys cannot excrete urine that is more acidic than about 5.0; in order to dilute this can of cola to an appropriate urinary pH, you'd need to produce approximately 30 litres of urine. So the body turns to its store of alkalizing minerals. If there aren't enough reserves of potassium and magnesium in the extracellular fluid, the calcium will be taken from the bone.

Some of the symptoms of acidosis are impaired cellular function, fatigue, weight gain, diminished immunity, inflammation, osteoporosis, premature aging, muscle loss, anxiety and irritability.

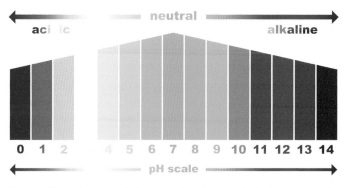

Cancer cells are known to thrive in acidity (low pH) but not in alkalinity (high pH). The presence of cancer cells makes the body even more acidic as they produce lactic acid. Therefore a diet high in alkaline foods like fruits and vegetables will raise blood pH levels and create an environment within the body that discourages cancer growth.

While limiting your intake of processed foods will help, even some nutritionally valid foods like fresh meat and dairy are very acidic. In other words, even nourishing, natural foods can contribute to the bone-sucking acidity of your body's pH….if you don't eat a balanced diet.

One simple method of testing the pH level in your body is the use of pH testing strips which are inexpensive and easy to use. Although this will give an indication into pH levels, this can only be assumed to be accurate at the time of testing.

How to maintain an ideal pH.

We would not for one minute suggest cutting out meat, cheese, eggs for example from your diet. While meat, eggs, and cheese are acidic, they are also nourishing for the body. These foods help build new cells and support your system under stress and chronic illness, growth, pregnancy, intense physical activity, etc. They are not to be confused with depleting acidic foods like sugar, factory farmed meat, or

Page 83

pasteurized dairy. In other words, these foods can be acidic, but you also need them to stay healthy.

The key is to eat enough alkaline foods to keep your pH balanced, while you eat those other nourishing (if acidic) foods. Drinking mineralized, alkaline water is one of the easiest and best ways to add alkalinity to your diet.

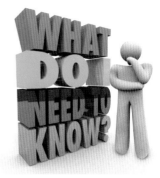

IN BRIEF

The pH of the body affects all cells, tissues, glands and organs.

A slightly alkaline pH of approximately 7.30-7.45 is required to maintain a healthy body.

The body ensures that blood remains within its healthy, slightly alkaline range.

Our blood achieves the pH balance by using important minerals from our organs, glands, tissues and bones if it is too acidic. A well balanced diet will help the blood to achieve its pH balance naturally.

Cancer cells are known to thrive in acidity but not in alkalinity.

Consuming a healthy balanced diet will encourage a raised blood pH level which is an environment that discourages cancer growth.

pH testing strips are easily purchased and inexpensive. They can be used as a daily guide to pH levels. However, testing of pH is a moment in time.

Water is essential for life and to maintain our health and therefore, it is important that we consume the correct amount. With all of the different types of water available and all of the hype that goes with each, it can be very easy to get confused about which types of water are really best for your health. It is understandable that there is also difficulty posed by the environmental concerns of bottled water against the dangerous chemicals found in tap water. The aim is to enable you to understand the options available to enable you to make the choice that is right for you and will benefit your health.

It is essential that we focus on the importance of fluid intake and the associated dangers of dehydration. Many people are not tuned into the required daily fluid intake the body needs to function at its optimum level. Alongside this, we are often guilty of ignoring the signs our body gives us that we are in need of fluid and are dehydrated.

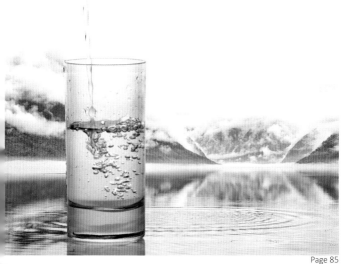

Water Consumption

Throughout a normal day the body is constantly losing water, primarily through urine and sweat. The health authorities commonly recommend fluid intake of 1.5 – 2 litres per day and advise that this fluid should predominantly comprise of water as it contains no sugar, calories or additives.

There is a silent and growing epidemic of chronic dehydration as a large number of the population do not drink enough water. So many people will suffer from this and are totally unaware. The body has its own ways of indicating that fluid is required. Thirst is one of the first signs that you need to drink more.

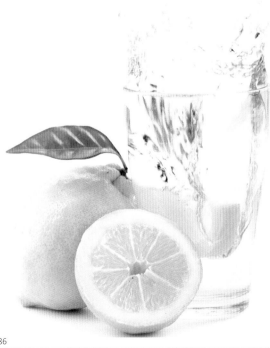

Another clear indicator as to how well you are hydrated is the colour of your urine. If you are in good health and are drinking sufficient, urine will be straw coloured and as dehydration sets in, urine will become progressively darker. Dark brown urine is a classic sign of severe dehydration and at this point, the lack of fluid intake will be having a real impact on the body's ability to function.

There are other commonly overlooked symptoms of chronic dehydration that most people are not aware of. Raising awareness of these will enable you to be more in tune with your body so that you know when your fluid intake is inadequate for your bodies' requirements.

Digestive disturbances such as heartburn and constipation, urinary tract infections, autoimmune disease such as chronic fatigue syndrome and multiple sclerosis, premature aging, high cholesterol and weight gain are all signs of chronic dehydration.

Types of Water – How your choice can make the difference

When it comes to water, there is more to choose from than simply tap versus bottled. We will explain this in further detail to enable you to make an informed decision about your water consumption and how it can impact on your health. It is common sense to do so.

Tap water is an obvious starting point. It is convenient and accessible to most people. However, as I'm sure you've heard, most tap water is contaminated with a host of pollutants that increase your risk of serious health problems. The practice of ensuring our tap water is 'safe' to consume, involves the addition of large amounts of poisonous chemicals to it. The long-term ingestion of these chemicals is not yet known although it could be the cause of a number of major health problems.

Liquid chlorine, aluminium sulphate and calcium hydroxide are just a few of the chemicals that are routinely added to our water supply. Once your water leaves the treatment plant, it travels through pipes that may have been underground for years. It would be almost impossible for this water to come out of our taps without any trace of contamination from something that we do not want to ingest. Over 300 man-made chemicals have been detected in British tap water in various quantities which is a concerning thought.

Brunel University in London conducted research into the condition of British water and what we are unknowingly consuming when we drink from the tap. This study focussed on prescription medications and British tap water. Almost half of the men and women in the UK take some form of regular prescribed medication. Due to the advances in the pharmaceutical industry, medications are more stable and last longer. This in turn, means that a percentage of these drugs remains unaltered through the sewage process and is able to re-enter the domestic water supply. Levels of anti-depressants, oestrogen from contraceptive pills and blood pressure medications are some of the commonly found drugs in the water that comes from the tap.

In view of the information as to

what our tap water contains, it may be a natural decision to start to drink bottled water to prevent unnecessary intake of harmful chemicals. However, it is now well known that approximately 30% of bottled water is actually just tap water which may or may not have received additional filtration. Evocative names and labels depicting idyllic rural scenes are used to convince the consumer that bottled water is the purest and safest water you could find. Bottled water companies will have to start to state on labels as to whether the water is from public water sources which will at least then mean that consumers are well informed and not being misled.

Another consideration as to whether bottled water is better is that plastic bottles contain a chemical called bisphenol A or BPA, which is a synthetic hormone disruptor that has been linked to serious health problems including prostate and breast cancer.

Some health conscious people have been misled into believing that distilled water is healthy for them. The problem with distilled water is that it is boiled and evaporated away from its dissolved minerals. The water then becomes acidic and seeks to balance itself by drawing minerals right out of your body. It will also draw out contaminants from the container it's stored in for this same reason. Further, any contaminant in the water that vaporizes at a lower temperature than the water such as volatile organic compounds, like disinfection by-products that are thousands of times as toxic as chlorine, will be condensed and actually concentrated in the finished distilled water. So what you end up with is water that contains even more dangerous contaminants than what you started with!

Distilled water should only be used for a short period of time and only for detoxification purposes as this type of water can help to draw toxins out of your body. Long term consumption of distilled water will most likely cause health problems.

Alkaline water is water that is less acidic than tap water. This means that it is rich in alkalizing compounds including calcium, silica, potassium, magnesium and bicarbonate.

We recommend drinking only natural mineral water, preferably from a recognised and established company. You should aim to be consuming natural mineral water that has a pH of 7 or above.

IN BRIEF

A daily intake of at least 1.5-2litres of water is required to enable the body to function.

Many people do not consume enough water and ignore signals of dehydration.

A good indication of hydration status is the colour of urine – darker coloured urine indicates a level of dehydration and that more fluids are required.

Tap water is contaminated with pollutants that increase the risk of developing health problems.

Glass bottled water is better than plastic bottles.

Approximately 30% of bottled water is actually tap water that may or may not have received additional filtration. So do your research.

There are many truly remarkable natural therapies that can be used in the fight against cancer. When you consider that progress has reportedly been made in orthodox cancer treatments, the numbers of those who are affected by cancer and will ultimately die because of this disease are at an all-time high. Therefore, we need to look to the effective natural methods instead of focussing on the cut-burn-poison approach which is so readily offered to patients after diagnosis.

Hemp oil is made from the flowering buds of the cannabis plant. Making the oil can be a skilled specific process and this potent but effective treatment is thought to have reversed cancer in thousands of cases. No clinical studies have been conducted on its effectiveness as it cannot be patented. Without patent, pharmaceutical companies are unable to recoup the millions it costs to conduct a study.

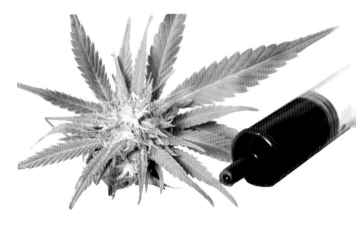

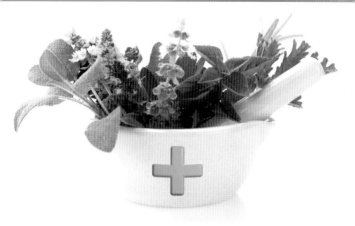

MMS (Miracle Mineral Solution) was discovered by an engineer, Jim Humble. He initially used this to reverse Malaria in South America and now claims that it will help to reverse 95% of all cancers. MMS is a common inexpensive mineral compound and is considered to be a safe cancer therapy. It is a highly diluted solution of chlorine dioxide and water which kills pathogens.

Gerson Natural Therapy is a natural option that activates the body's extraordinary ability to heal itself with no damaging side effects. Dr Gerson believed that cancer would not survive in a body that had a well-balanced, fully functioning liver. He discovered that the majority of cancers could be reversed by dietary changes. This focusses on eating a vegan diet (no meat or dairy) coupled with low salt intake and drinking freshly juiced fruits and vegetables ten times a day. Coffee enemas were recommended as part of the treatment for pain relief and detoxification.

Antineoplastins were discovered by Dr Stanislaw Burzynski. He is recognised internationally for the discovery and development of options in the fight against cancer with biologically active peptides. He discovered that people who developed cancer were missing these peptides in their urine and blood compared to those who do not have cancer that have these peptides. Since 1967, Dr Burzynski has worked from his clinic in Texas and has treated over 50 types of cancer effectively. He has had most success with cancers of the ovaries, lungs, prostrate, colon, head and neck, breast and non-Hodgkin's lymphoma. He has possibly discovered the most successful FDA approved drug therapy for cancer ever. His antineoplastins (which have no toxic side effects) significantly outperform any chemotherapy treatment making it one of the best alternative cancer therapies.

Pancreatic enzymes were used by Dr William Kelley to develop a highly effective natural protocol for treating advanced cancers. He did this with pancreatic enzymes and other nutritional substances. In his second year of Medical school, Dr Gonzalez met Dr Kelly and spent five years researching Dr Kelley's thousands of patient records. After personally interviewing many of these patients and finding them in good health, Dr Gonzalez realised that something very important was occurring.

Today, Dr Gonzalez has refined and improved on Dr Kelley's original discoveries, giving each patient an individualised diet with supplements and large quantities of enzymes. Coffee enemas, juice fasts and liver flushes are also incorporated for detoxification purposes.

Salve treatment is a salve made from bloodroot and is used as a treatment for skin cancers. Some other names for this are Black Salve, Indian Mud or Compound X. Bloodroot salve works by drawing the tumours out through the skin whilst healing underneath as the mass falls out.

Energy healing is done by specially trained practitioners who project energy known in Chinese medicine as Chi or Qi. A sonogram is used so that cancer tumours can be seen to dissolve whilst the therapy is being delivered.

LifeOne is a therapy which has the active ingredients including selenium methionine, green tea extract, quercetin, turmeric, resveratrol, diindolymethane, versicolor, coriolus and chrysin. LifeOne has had clinical trials with cancer patients in Mexico and

Venezuela. Trials show that LifeOne has been able to help to reverse an extremely wide variety of cancer cell types including two types of breast cancer, colon, prostate, cervical and ovarian cancer as well as acute promyelocytic leukaemia.

Alkaline Diet is based on the notion that the metabolism of cancer cells has a very narrow pH tolerance and if you are able to interfere with the metabolism of cancer cells, theoretically you are then able to stop cancer in its tracks. The proposed alkaline therapy has been developed to normalise the intracellular pH of the cancer while increasing the pH of cancer cells to a range above 7.5. According to published research, it is at that pH that cell death is experienced. The alkaline diet which is primarily plant-based avoids sugar, dairy, wheat and other high-gluten grains. There is an emphasis on fresh vegetables and juices and this all serves to change the body's intracellular pH.

Cesium Chloride is the most alkaline mineral salt in nature and is non-toxic. It has been used as a medical treatment since the 1800's and has been used to successfully treat cancer patients since the 1980's. It is also known to remove pain caused by cancerous tumours and would be a good addition to those following the Alkaline Diet.

Essiac Tea is a long proven method of helping to treat cancer, going as far back to 1920's. Named by Rene Caisse, the tea consists of four main herbs that grow in the wilderness of Ontario, Canada. The original formula is believed to have its roots from the native Canadian Ojibway Indians.

The four main ingredients are burdock root, slippery elm inner bark, sheep sorrel and rhubarb root. Whilst the basic components of Essiac are well known, the exact proportions of the herbs are a matter of much speculation. It is important that the patient is concerned with both the quality of the herbs, and the quality of the processing. Sheep sorrel is the main cancer killing herb in Essiac tea.

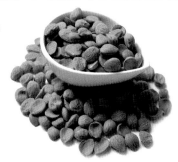

Laetrile (vitamin B17) reacts with cancer cell enzymes to form hydrogen cyanide that helps to destroy the cancer cells on contact. Incredibly, it manages to do this without destroying the surrounding healthy cells.

Iscador is made from certain fermented extracts of the European mistletoe plant and has been used across Europe since approximately 1920. There are approximately 5,000 case studies focussing on the success of the use of Iscador to treat cancer. Two scientific reviews demonstrate the following findings in support for the use of Iscador therapy.

*After a period of approximately 3 years, the survival rate for patients with skin cancer who took Iscador was over 75% compared to over

65% for those not taking it.

*Over 70% of bronchial cancer patients taking Iscador were living after a 4 year period compared to only below 40% of those not taking it.

*An over 80% five year survival rate for women with cervical cancer if they followed treatment of surgery, radiotherapy and Iscador compared to over 65% for those who only had radiation.

*A significantly larger number of women with breast cancer treated with Iscador were doing well after approximately 10 years in comparison to those who did not have Iscador treatment.

IN BRIEF

There are a vast amount of natural therapies available which are known to help in the fight against cancer.

The natural remedy approach can be adopted alone, or alongside orthodox cancer treatments.

The above therapies are simply a suggestion of what is available and is not an exhaustive list.

These therapies can be used as stand-alone options or combined together if suitable for the individual.

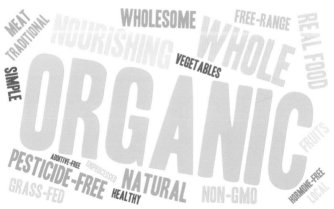

Oxygen to Fight Cancer: What is Oxygen Therapy?

Oxygen is required for cell growth in the body. However, cancer cells are different and have a unique and dangerous metabolism which means that they do not depend on oxygen like normal cells do. The way they metabolize and create energy for living and multiplication is unique and specific and high levels of oxygen are toxic to cancer cells. Whilst normal cells thrive on oxygen, cancer cells do not – they prefer glucose (sugar). Flooding the body with oxygen has the potential to slow the growth of cancer cells and can trigger cell death mechanisms within them.

A German doctor named Otto Warburg was awarded the Nobel Prize in 1931 for his research proving that cancer cells use a form of non-oxygen metabolism to survive.

Oxygen provides far less fuel for cancer cells than glucose (only 2 energy molecules instead of 36 with sugar). Therefore, filling your body with more oxygen is an effective and safe method to help to fight cancer.

There are different oxygen therapies you might consider s below.

Hyperbaric oxygen is a mechanism that increases the pressure of oxygen forcing more into the blood and tissues. This involves breathing pure oxygen in a pressurised room. Under such conditions it is possible for the lungs to gather up to three times more oxygen than they would if pure oxygen was used in normal air pressure.

Oxygen to Fight Cancer: What is Oxygen Therapy?

Hyperbaric oxygen appears to significantly reduce the side effects of radiotherapy and would appear to diminish the unpleasant side effects of tissue damage and inflammation caused by radiation.

For those struggling with lymphoedema following breast cancer requiring lymph node surgery, hyperbaric oxygen therapy helps to reduce swelling and pain and has been shown to soften the damaged tissue.

Oxygen flooding is increasing oxygenation through the use of peroxide and ozone. The two substances are super-charged with oxygen and deliver a high-impact yield. This process involves the delivery of peroxide and ozone through the veins in your body or by removing blood and oxygenating it before it is then returned to your body.

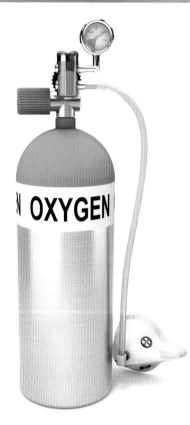

Using oxygen therapy to help to kill cancer is practiced around the world with some excellent results. Choose your practitioner wisely through the International Oxidative Medicine Association (IOMA) – and still check them out. Always consult with your healthcare practitioner beforehand to determine if this option is right for you.

Oxygen to Fight Cancer: What is Oxygen Therapy?

IN BRIEF

Cancer cells differ in how they metabolise and create energy for multiplication compared to normal cells in the body.

High levels of oxygen are toxic to cancer cells.

Flooding the body with oxygen can slow the growth of cancer cells and cause cell death.

Hyperbaric oxygen therapy increases the pressure of oxygen and forces higher levels into the bloodstream and tissues.

Oxygen flooding uses peroxide and ozone to increase oxygen levels in the body.

Research is needed to ensure that you select your practitioner wisely.

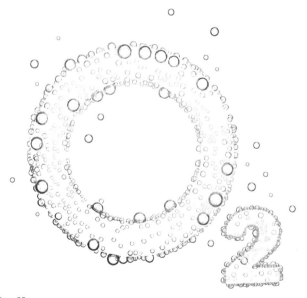

The health benefits of exercise extend far beyond management of weight as research shows that regular physical activity can help to reduce the risk of developing disease including cancer and heart disease.

Inactivity is actually as much of a health risk to the body as smoking is, although little emphasis is placed on this in relation to smoking and disease onset. Alongside the protection against disease, regular exercise can improve mood, reduce depression and assist with management of stress. Therefore, maintaining a level of regular physical activity will help to create a feeling of well-being and positive outlook whilst reducing risk of disease.

The benefits of exercise on the cardiovascular system are well known. However, there is now evidence to show that physical activity reduces the risk of developing breast, bowel and womb cancer. Hormone levels in the body, such as insulin and oestrogen are altered during exercise. It is known that oestrogen fuels the development of breast and womb cancer and

therefore by reducing oestrogen through exercise, the risk of developing these cancers is also reduced. It is estimated that keeping active could prevent over 3,000 cases of cancer yearly in the United Kingdom.

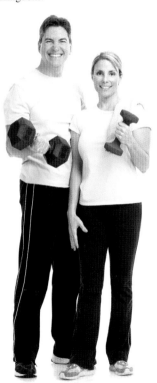

By keeping active, food moves through the bowel at a quicker rate which prevents harmful chemicals in food damaging the lining of the bowel. This chemical damage can lead to the development of cancer and therefore, maintaining a level of exercise can help to prevent bowel cancer.

Research has shown that when comparing levels of sedentary behaviour, those with the highest levels were at a greater risk of developing colon, endometrial and lung cancers. This risk increased with each 2 hour increase in sitting time. This demonstrates that one period of activity per day is of no benefit if the rest of that day is spent sitting. Maintaining some level of activity throughout the day will assist in creating a balance between the unhealthy and healthy hormones, which in turn will ensure a healthier body.

A commonly asked question is what level of exercise is advised following a diagnosis of cancer and whilst undergoing treatments for cancer. This is specific to each individual and also will depend on the amount of exercise you were doing prior to diagnosis.

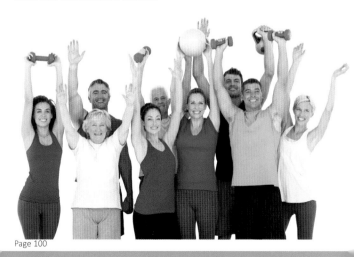

The key is to remain active. This will promote a feeling of well-being and will encourage the positive mind-set that is crucial to fighting cancer. In turn, it will also reduce the risk of developing further cancers. So any type of physical activity will be beneficial and will support your chosen journey.

You must also listen to your body. It will tell you when you may have done too much and rest is required. A sensible approach to any physical exercise is recommended. Find something that you enjoy and can maintain as part of your treatment plan.

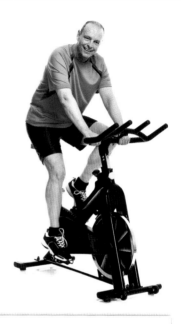

IN BRIEF

Regular physical activity can reduce the risk of developing diseases such as cancer and heart disease.

Regular exercise also can reduce the risk of developing breast, bowel and womb cancers.

Exercise at any level will promote a positive mind set and will reduce stress and anxiety.

Listen to your body.

Find something that you can work into your day and that more importantly, you enjoy.

With or without cancer, exercise has many advantages to your health.

On a daily basis and often unknowingly, we are exposing ourselves to toxins that are damaging our health and are known contributing factors to disease. Whilst people are becoming more educated on issues related to healthy living, there are many areas of our everyday lives that are overlooked and could be the source of toxin exposure.

Our bodies constantly absorb from our surroundings. The skin is the largest organ of the body and is a porous, absorbent network of glands that interacts with external elements. Therefore, our skin will absorb whatever is applied to it. Without possibly realising, we are exposed to more toxic chemicals from the

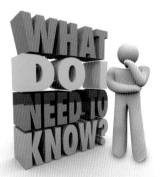

environment than we ever have been.

We are applying these potential cancer causing chemicals – with no consideration as to how they will affect our health over time.

The carcinogens that our bodies are exposed to may cause cells to divide at a faster than normal rate which increase the possibility of DNA alterations. Carcinogenic substances do not cause cancer in each of us all of the time. This is because the cancer causing potential of carcinogens depends on the levels of exposure along with how long this exposure has occurred for along with genetic makeup. So for each individual, the effect of exposure to carcinogens will differ. To reduce the possibility of cancer developing as a result of the carcinogens we expose ourselves to, it is essential to have an understanding of what everyday products contain these toxic chemicals.

DEODORANTS

The use of most antiperspirants exposes the body to aluminium which is a neurotoxin as this is one of the sweat blocking ingredients used. The use of antiperspirants also

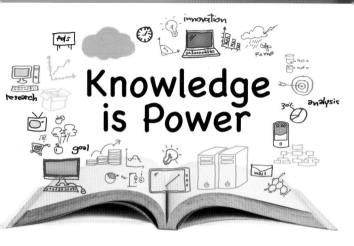

restricts the natural processes of the bodies' sweat glands and as a result, causes entrapment of toxins within the body. Aluminium can be absorbed by the skin and mimics oestrogen which promotes the growth of breast cancer. Parabens are also a common ingredient in deodorant and they also mimic oestrogen and are therefore linked to the development of breast cancer. It is recommended that natural deodorant is used instead to prevent unnecessary exposure to these cancer causing chemicals. Chemical-free deodorants kill the bacteria which causes odour at the source rather than blocking pores and preventing sweat glands from functioning. There are many natural, organic alternatives available.

AIR FRESHENERS

Most houses, cars and workplaces will use air fresheners and over time, these have replaced the traditional methods of maintaining a pleasant environment such as potpourris and natural pomanders. Common chemicals found in most air fresheners used are acetaldehyde and benzaldehyde which are both known carcinogens. Alongside these chemicals, petroleum-based solvents and fragrances are used which create a potent carcinogenic that many chose to have in their homes. Consider a natural, chemical free alternative such as essential oils or the use of citrus fruits and spices to create the same effect whilst reducing exposure to toxic substances.

CANDLES

Candles are a product that can be found in most homes. However, candles made from paraffin wax release carcinogenic fumes when lit. Therefore, a regular habit of lighting candles around the home will result in exposure to these carcinogens. A safe alternative is to use natural beeswax candles instead.

SUNSCREEN

The damage caused by exposure to the sun has resulted in an increased use of sunscreens to prevent premature ageing and skin cancer. Ironically, it is now the sunscreen that is used to protect from UV rays that is a potential cancer causing substance. One common ingredient in most sunscreens is zinc oxide which is known to produce free radicals which can damage DNA

and result in the development of cancerous cells. Look for a natural alternative but more importantly, reduce your exposure to the sun's harmful rays. Sun exposure is beneficial in sensible amounts as it provides the body with much needed vitamin D. Too much exposure is damaging and therefore a common sense approach is needed.

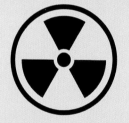

EXPOSURE TO EMFR (Electromagnetic Field Radiation)

Electromagnetic fields arise whenever electrical energy is used. It is known that over a period of time, exposure to levels of EMFR can have detrimental effects to the human body. The damage caused will depend on the frequency of the radiation emitted. With the advances in modern technology such as mobile phone networks, Wi-Fi signals and household appliances it is simply not possible to reduce exposure to EMFR to zero. However, it is this exposure to low frequency EMFR that is more controversial as symptoms can be inconspicuous and may only manifest over a long time when damage has already occurred. Therefore it is essential that steps are taken to minimise the EMFR the body is exposed to. Smart meters for example are accepted readily into people's homes to enable them to give control over energy use. What isn't advertised is the fact that these meters emit short bursts of microwave radiation throughout the day which in turn, can result in health problems such as migraines, dizziness and anxiety to name a few. Be aware of the hazards in and around your home in relation to EMFR exposure and take action to ensure that health risks related to EMFR exposure are reduced.

HAIR CARE PRODUCTS

Hair shampoo and conditioner is used often with little consideration as to what it contains. Very few people read the labels on such well used, common products. We are naturally more interested in the larger print on the product and what it promises it will do to our hair. However, chemicals such as polyethylene glycol (PEG), cocamide DEA and sodium lauryl sulfate will be found in most hair care products. These chemicals, when used together have been shown to be carcinogenic. The basis of cocamide DEA is actually coconut oil which is altered to modify it into an unnatural and toxic

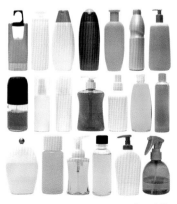

form. This chemical is simply added to these products to thicken and as a foaming agent. So the small print on hair care products needs attention to ensure exposure to carcinogens is reduced.

CLEANING AGENTS

Cleaning products are loaded with toxic chemicals including silica. These products are sprayed on surfaces in most homes without a second thought for what they contain and more importantly what damage they could do. Most cleaning routines will involve the inhalation and direct skin contact with a multitude of toxic chemicals that are known carcinogens. This exposure occurs daily and therefore it is essential to switch to natural chemical free cleaning products to eliminate this exposure.

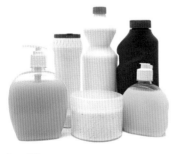

COSMETICS

Common sense would tell us that what we apply to our skin should be as clean as the food we ingest although for most people this is not the case. Even in the smallest amounts, the chemicals applied to our skin which are commonly found in many cosmetics, can have a tremendous impact on our health. Almost 1 in 5 commonly used cosmetic products will contain a formaldehyde-releaser which is a compound that releases formaldehyde as it decomposes. The reason this is used commonly in cosmetics is that they are an antifungal and antimicrobial preservative. This irritant can be found in nail products, eyelash adhesives hair gels and hair colourant to name a few. To put this into context, formaldehyde is used in the production of paper, plywood and fertiliser. This serves as a stark reminder as to how disconnected we are from what we put in and on our bodies. There are many online sites that list the least harmful cosmetics and those to avoid at all costs. This is a useful way to change your product choice and eliminates the need to decipher the ingredient list on all of the products you use.

By choosing wisely, you can reduce your exposure to harmful chemicals that can lead to cancer development. Please remember that whatever you chose for yourself should also be suitable for others. Children are not little adults. On a daily basis they are exposed to higher levels of toxins in air, water, food and personal products. Children's organ systems are immature and are therefore less capable of defending chemical assaults and any early damage can result in disease development later in life.

So in making better choices regarding the products you use on yourself, your children and within the home you can avoid exposure to dangerous chemicals that are known carcinogenics. Simple switches to safer products and having a greater awareness of what your products contain will have a huge impact on your health. This is just a short list to provide an example of what you may currently use with suggestions as to how you can change to ensure you do not compromise your health.

IN BRIEF

Many people are unaware of the daily toxin exposure caused by products used on the body or in the home.

The skin is the largest organ in the body and interacts with external elements.

The carcinogens that our bodies are exposed to may cause cells to divide at a faster than normal rate which increase the possibility of DNA alterations.

It is essential to have an understanding as to what products contain chemicals that may be harmful to your health.

Familiarise yourself with the labels on the products you use every day and what ingredients you need to avoid.

Remember that for each individual, the effect of exposure to carcinogens will differ depending on a number of factors.

Look into exchanging your current products for chemical free, safe versions.

Seek recipes for homemade skin and cleaning products for peace of mind as to what ingredients they contain.

Ensure the changes are made for the whole household especially children to prevent exposure to chemicals that may in time result in development of disease.

The Hunza community. An example of the power of apricot kernels.

The Hunza Valley is a mountainous region in Pakistan. The people live off the land and their diet consists mostly of the plants indigenous to the area and cultivated fruits and vegetables. Wholegrains grown in the absence of pesticides or synthetic fertilisers alongside a small amount of meat, cheese and yoghurt are also consumed by the Hunza community. The people are cheerful, healthy and full of life, look youthful and hardly ever succumb to illness.

The life expectancy of the average Hunza is 120 years which is unheard of in any other part of the world. The women can conceive well into their 60's and it is rare for the Hunza people to develop tumours.

How is this possible? How do they stay healthy? What are their secrets?

The saying 'you are what you eat' is the secret behind the health of the Hunza people. Rather than living to eat, they eat to live. They have two meals a day; a rich breakfast in the morning followed by dinner after sunset. Moreover, they only eat natural food products such as fruits, vegetables, grains, milk, and cheese and there are no chemicals or additives in their meals. It is true to say that in the West we lead a totally different lifestyle. However, we can learn from the lifestyle of the Hunza.

There is no such thing as cancer in Hunza.

According to research, apricots of the Hunza Valley are said to be the

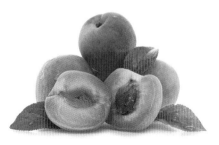

key behind the absence of tumours. Hunzas eat large amounts of the fruit which is rich in Amygdalin (vitamin B-17). Amygdalin is widely known for its anticancer properties. They crush the kernels and use these in cooking. None of the apricot fruit is wasted. Once a year for a period of two to four months, Hunzas take a break from their regular diet and solely live on the juice of dried apricots. It is an old tradition that they still follow during the time when apricots are unripe. Scientists agree that it contributes to their amazing health.

Alongside their diet, there is practically zero pollution in the air, earth and water. The water the

people use for cooking, drinking and bathing is snow run-off from the Himalayas. The water therefore contains no fluoride or chlorine. There is no toxic waste from manufacturing or harmful chemicals used within the home or on the body.

Children and adults alike are physically active all day long. The food they eat is in moderation and the Hunza people only take in what is needed. All of life's basic needs are covered and there is no need for more. These people are healthy and content.

Free from disease as a result of their lifestyle habits.

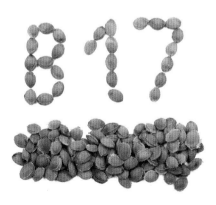

Caffeine is an alkaloid that the coffee plant uses to kill bugs, which eat its' seeds. The coffee plant also uses caffeine in the coffee pods to kill surrounding plants, so the coffee plant can attain more sunlight and grow larger. Caffeine is a pesticide, which causes genetic termination in living cells that come into contact with it.

MRI images taken before and after 1 cup of coffee containing caffeine have shown a decrease in blood flow to the brain by over 40%. When the blood flow reduction was measured exactly, it was actually over 50% less blood flow to the brain, after just one small cup of coffee containing caffeine.

Brain imaging studies of chronic coffee drinkers showed they presented the same degradation of their brains as chronic alcoholics, cigarette smokers and Parkinson's patients.

Caffeine can cause an urge to move ones' bowels because this is one way the body tries to eliminate poison from the system. The sudden urge to "poo" after drinking caffeinated coffee is one of the body's defence mechanisms to poison.

Caffeine increases energy via the human fight or flight metabolic response, because the body is afraid of the caffeine based poison. Caffeinated coffee doesn't give energy; it removes it from the body. The energy a person feels when they drink caffeine is the body going into overdrive because it is a poison and all poisons activate an energy release in the body. Caffeine removes energy from the system, leaving the person progressively more and more exhausted each day that passes, therefore setting up the world's most dangerous energy stimulation addiction.........caffeinated coffee dependence for energy.

When measured, 1 cup of caffeinated coffee activated the fight and flight response for over 2 weeks, even though no other caffeine was consumed after that 1 cup of coffee. One cup of caffeinated coffee poisons the body for more than 2 weeks, on a decreasing scale.

Caffeine can be the cause of an enlarged prostate, high anxiety, insomnia, depression, birth defects, pain syndromes, unnatural breathing patterns, brain damage, hyperactivity, learning disorders (from the brain damage) behaviour disorders, fatigue, certain types of cancer, Crohns, IBS, colitis, carpel tunnel, ulcers, low iron, heart disease, headaches, PMS, increased incidence of muscle and tendon injury, joint pain, heart attack, stroke,TIA's (mini strokes)...and that's a short list.

Caffeine may contribute to fat gain and cellulite because by triggering the body's flight or fight system (which any poison or threat does)

this eventually changes the body's primary fuel source requirement to one of fat. When the body is threatened, it prefers fat as its' primary fuel source, over sugar or protein. Constant activation of the body's fight or flight system (via the daily ingestion of caffeine poison) aids in a metabolic shift to fat storage and fat conservation, because again the body prefers fat as a fuel source when fighting any toxic intruder..... Because fat contains 9 calories per gram for the fight, as opposed to 4 calories per gram housed by sugar and protein. Welcome to the land of caffeine

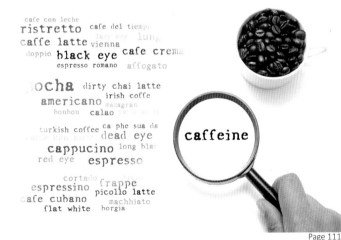

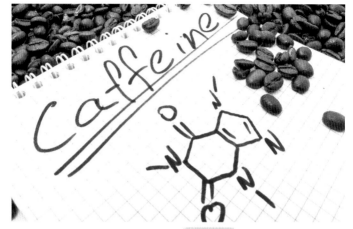

induced fat gain, weight gain and cellulite. Caffeine also destroys muscle, as the body purposely flushes muscle, when it's poisoned, to facilitate additional fat storage.

Caffeine blocks iron absorption, contributing to the vast majority of anaemia today. The entire threat of caffeine in general includes caffeine teas, chocolates, caffeine based energy drinks, caffeine based pre work out drinks and over 2000 over the counter and prescription medications that PURPOSELY include caffeine.

IN BRIEF

Caffeine is a pesticide, which causes genetic termination in living cells that come into contact with it.

Caffeine is known to decrease blood flow to the brain.

Caffeine can have similar damaging effects to cigarettes and alcohol intake.

The urge to defecate after consuming coffee illustrates that caffeine is a poison which the body then attempts to eliminate.

Caffeine can be a contributory factor of insomnia, depression, heart disease and certain cancers to name a few.

Lung cancer is possibly the UK's biggest cancer killer with over 95 people per day dying from lung cancer each year. This is more than breast cancer, bladder cancer and prostate cancer combined. Lung cancer accounts for approximately 6% of all deaths in the UK.

Unlike heart disease, there is a widespread recognition that tobacco is by far the most common cause of lung cancer. Over 80% of lung cancer cases are among smokers. Men who smoke are up to 20 times more likely and women who smoke are over 10 times more likely to develop lung cancer than non-smokers. Smokers are not just harming themselves – thousands of deaths each year have been attributed to passive smoking.

So, as a non-smoker, you have over a 20 % chance of developing lung cancer if there is regular exposure to cigarette smoke.

The warning labels on cigarette packets are everywhere now but for a long time, the link between smoking and lung cancer appears to have been supressed by powerful interest groups much as the relationship between certain foods and other leading killers is supressed today. For example, in the 1980's, Phillip Morris, the nation's leading cigarette manufacturer launched the notorious white coat project. The corporation hired doctors to publish ghost written studies attempting to negate links between second hand smoke and lung disease. These papers cherry picked various scientific reports to conceal and

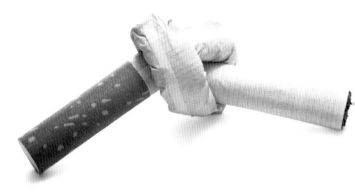

distort the damning evidence of the dangers of passive smoking. This whitewashing, coupled with the tobacco industry's clever marketing campaigns, including cartoon like adverts helped to hook generations onto their products. If despite all of the evidence and warnings you are currently a smoker, the most important step you can take is to stop. It makes sense. The benefits of quitting are immediate. According to the American Cancer Society, after just 20 minutes of not smoking your heart rate and blood pressure drops. Within just a few weeks, your blood circulation and lung function improve and within a few months

the sweeper cells that help to clean the lungs, remove mucous and reduce the risk of infection. Within a whole year of quitting, your smoking relating risk of coronary heart disease becomes half that of current smokers.

The human body possesses the miraculous ability to heal itself as long as we do not keep reinjuring it. Simple dietary changes may help to roll back the damage caused by the carcinogens in tobacco smoke. It is important to understand the toxic effects of cigarettes on the lungs as tobacco smoke contains chemicals that weaken the body's immune system making it more susceptible to disease and handicapping its ability to destroy cancer cells. We have already looked into a compromised immune system and it is essential that you do everything in your power to ensure that you are no longer compromising your immune system. By stopping smoking, it will enable the immune system to become stronger, not weaker.

IN BRIEF

Lung cancer is possibly the UK's biggest cancer killer.

More than 95 people die daily from this disease.

Over 75% of those diagnosed with lung cancer are smokers.

Passive smoking and regular exposure to cigarette smoke results in over a 20% chance of a lung cancer diagnosis.

The benefits of stopping smoking are seen almost immediately.

Heart rate and blood pressure reduce after only 20 minutes of stopping smoking.

After 24 hours your lungs start to clear.

The body is nicotine free after only 2 days of not smoking and after 3 days, energy levels increase.

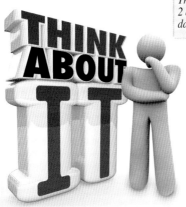

Conclusion

Receiving the news that you have cancer is life changing and can trigger a range of emotions in each individual. Life will never be the same again – the journey you take to fight this disease will change you and your outlook on life forever. This does not have to be a negative – the journey will teach you many things about yourself and will show you how strong you can be when faced with illness.

You may feel angry, anxious about your future or that you have no control over what is happening. Conventional treatments will be discussed with medical professionals which may cause more turmoil about whether you are taking the right path. You may feel pressure from family, friends and healthcare professionals which can be overwhelming. Time is also an additional pressure as to ensure the best outcome, treatment decisions have to be made quickly to ensure that the cancer does not spread. The complex decisions come at an already stressful time and you may struggle to process the amount of information you receive.

This guide is written to enable you to begin taking control over what is happening. At a time when you may feel like your options are limited, it was our intention when writing this guide to demonstrate how you can adapt your lifestyle and use some of the many natural options available. In turn this will alleviate some of the anxiety and lack of empowerment that your diagnosis may be causing you.

This guide illustrates that the path you chose is individual to you. You are in control and can make small changes which will have a great impact going forward. You may choose some of the options suggested but feel that others are not for you. You can tailor your own plan to ensure that you gain the most benefit. Ultimately you need to empower your immune system to enable it to function to its optimum level and the guide will enable you to make choices that will help with this.

The journey you are taking will not be smooth. The intention is not to gloss over the true, harsh impact that a battle with cancer has on individuals and their loved ones. There will always be bumps in the road and hurdles for you to overcome. Nothing worthwhile in life comes easily.

You need to take control and make your own decisions. This journey is about you and ensuring that you do everything in your power to fight this disease.

A positive mind set is your best weapon coupled with knowledge and common sense. Always remember that cancer is a disease of the body that has a compromised immune system. So, empowerment of the immune system coupled with our endocannabinoid system is necessary for the human body to be in the best position to fight cancer. Remain focussed on your goal and remember that you, like many others are more than capable of reversing this disease. Fact.

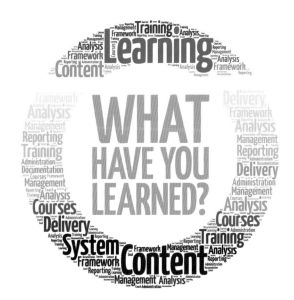

Points to remember

☑ Cancer does not lead to imminent death.

☑ Empowerment of the Immune System is paramount

☑ A positive mindset is vital for yourself and those around you.

☑ Feed your body to help fight the disease;
do not feed the disease.

☑ Cannabinoids are needed to empower our
endocannabinoid system

☑ Stay focussed at all times; realise that YOU can
make a difference

☑ 1000,s of people reverse this disease every day worldwide.

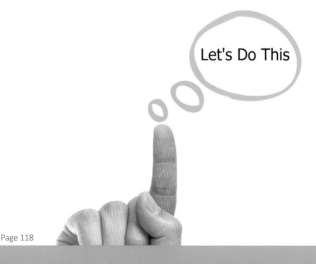

Let's Do This

Mr Mohammed Razaq

Fighting cancer and winning May 2018
Preston, Lancashire

"This book will help everyone, I highly recommend it"
★★★★★

I was initially diagnosed with kidney cancer in early 2016. The size of the tumour was such that unfortunately the cancerous kidney had to be removed. I was told that this would hopefully be curative and would require no further treatment. However, on my follow up scan a few months later I was given the news that the cancer had reappeared. Worse still, it had spread. At this point I was told that my prognosis was terminal and that in time the disease would overcome me. Two years on and after a roller coaster of a ride, I feel better now than I have done at any time since being diagnosed. Cancer is a shock to the system and the devastating effects aren't limited to just the victim or just to do with physical and mental health. It affects your livelihood, your relationships and it affects all those close to you. To give yourself the best chance of overcoming cancer you need to have a holistic approach and not just rely on conventional medical interventions. Support from family and friends is essential to make life bearable, to keep your mind occupied and prevent negative thoughts.

A drastic change in diet will give your body the right kind of foods and certainly reduce those foods which are instinctively bad for you.

Alternative and natural options will give your immune system a boost and help you get plenty of rest.

Perhaps most importantly, my advice would be to do some research. You will be surprised to learn what else is out there and how effective it can be.

That's my experience - good luck and I hope my advice will be of some help. Remember to stay positive and focused throughout. A positive mind set is paramount. The book Cancer and Common Sense is an easy to understand book that really helps and will benefit everyone who reads it.

Mark Clements
Liverpool
Reversing cancer since 2009 and living life to the full.

"The book "Cancer and Common Sense" is a must read for any person fighting CANCER I highly recommend it"

★★★★★

I was diagnosed with lung cancer on April 1st 2009 and was informed that this had spread to the lymph nodes in my chest. I felt like my world was falling apart with my first thought being for my wife and 5 children.

On 14th May 2009 I commenced 3 months of chemotherapy and radiotherapy which quickly took its toll on my body. I lost almost 5 stone within 12 months. I was given a 3 month terminal prognosis.

By 2012, I had suffered with pneumonia twice. It was during the same year that I decided to look into natural remedies and how they may benefit me. I started using 'NATURAL PLANT OIL' and was able to discontinue the 36 pharmaceutical drugs I had been prescribed.

By 2014, my body was feeling and looking better. This continued on into 2015 when I felt like my mind, body and soul were much stronger. On 31st March 2016, I returned for my routine scan results to be informed that my tumour had reduced in size by 75%. Although my battle is ongoing, I am living proof that cancer is by no means a death sentence.

A positive mind-set has been the key to my success in the battle against cancer. This, alongside the natural therapies I have adopted into my lifestyle have ensured that I have been alive for much longer than the medical profession anticipated.

Empowerment of the immune system is paramount. Without my wife and children I would not be here today. Here's to many more years helping people to win their battle with cancer.